Macular Degeneration

"This book is an excellent reference source for those afflicted with macular degeneration, their families and friends. . . . Not only is this a comprehensive resource, but more importantly, the positive and uplifting spirit of the book will help to overcome the sense of fear and isolation experienced by many people diagnosed with macular degeneration."
— **Chip Goehring, President**
American Macular Degeneration Foundation

"This book will be a real spirit-lifter for people with visual impairments, our families and friends . . . It gives us what we need most— information about the equipment, organizations, possible treatments, support, coping techniques, and other resources that will help us lead happy, busy and productive lives despite our vision loss . . . I wish this book had existed when I received my diagnosis of Stargardt's!" — **Judy Schnitzer, activist and member of the Board,**
Macular Degeneration Foundation

Dedication

To Jacque, Ruth and Carl for the
generous sharing of their talents

Ordering Information

Macular Degeneration

Living Positively with Vision Loss

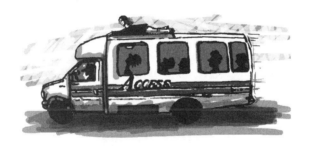

Betty Wason

with James J. McMillan, M.D.

PUBLISHERS

Hunter House Inc., Publishers
P.O. Box 2914
Alameda CA 94501-0914

Library of Congress Cataloging-in-Publication Data

Wason, Betty, 1912–
Macular degeneration : living positively with vision loss /
Betty Wason, with James J. McMillan.
p. cm.
Includes bibliographical references and index.
ISBN 0-89793-239-0 (paper). — ISBN 0-89793-240-4 (cloth)
1. Retinal degeneration—Popular works. I. McMillan, James J. II. Title.
RE661.D3W37 1998
617.7'35—dc21 98–42145
CIP

Project credits

Cover Design: Jil Weil Designs, Oakland	Book Design: *Qalagraphia*
Project Editor: Kiran Rana	Production Coordinator: Wendy Low
Copy Editor: Mali Apple	Proofreader: Lee Rappold
Marketing: Susan Markey, Corrine Sahli	Publicity: Marisa Spatafore
Customer Support: Christina Sverdrup, Joel Irons	
Order Fulfillment: A & A Quality Shipping Services	
Publisher: Kiran S. Rana	

Printed and Bound by Publishers Press, Salt Lake City, UT
Manufactured in the United States of America

9 8 7 6 5 4 3 2   First Edition

Contents

Acknowledgments vi

Foreword by Dr. James J. McMillan ix

Introduction 1

A Special Message to Families and Friends 4

1   How It Began for Me 6

2   The Mystery of the Eyes 17

3   About Eye Doctors 28

4   Symptoms, Risk Factors, and Treatments 40

5   A Vast Network of Services 59

6   Making Your Home Life Easier and Safer 75

7   Dealing with Stress 92

8   Diet and Exercise 110

9   Helpers Are Everywhere 134

10 The Wonders of Technology 146

11 Recreation Is Good for the Soul 160

12 Keep Your Spirits High and Your Kite Soaring 175

Resources 188

Notes 227

Glossary 232

Index 237

Acknowledgments

Naively, I thought in the very beginning that I could write this book by myself, because I have been a writer all my life. But that was when I could still read some large print. It didn't take long before the distortion of letters got worse and the glare of my computer screen began to bother me.

I was on the lookout for an assistant and found Holly Thomas through a friend. Holly and I together worked out a strong book proposal and wrote query letters to agents and publishers.

About the time Holly decided she couldn't afford to volunteer any longer, I put ads in several community papers to find replacements. Through these ads and through word of mouth, I found an amazing number of other volunteers.

My next-door neighbor Kali Rose had noticed me through my window pounding at my keyboard day after day, and she ended up taking on the two jobs of editorial assistant and professional advisor. We got along so well that she remained as my assistant until the book was published. Kali worked with me to revise the original book proposal, and about this time I met Alistair Black, an English professor, and he went over the new book proposal as a copy editor. There also arose a need for a filing system, and my friend Ruth Wilson, also an English teacher, came to the fore.

In the fall of 1997, my friend Georgia Kravitz decided to find me press coverage. She suggested to the *Seattle Times* columnist Terry McDermott that he write a story about my ambitious project. Terry was interested and on Thanksgiving Day his article appeared, mentioning my need for volunteers.

Jacque Blix had read Terry's article, and later on she became a vital copy editor who came on a daily basis. She and her husband coauthored the book *Getting a Life,* published recently by Viking.

For further assistance, I advertised in the classifieds of neighborhood weeklies and received many replies. One was a young man named Tad Wolff who had exactly the qualities I needed: computer skills and literary aspirations, as well as patience and loyalty.

Meantime, my vision became so blurred that I could not use the computer and had to write chapter drafts in longhand. Tad and Kali could be counted on to translate my scrawled words when scarcely anyone else could, and with both I could talk out my editorial changes as they skillfully made revisions on the computer.

About the time I met Kali, Ginette Perkins at the Washington Association for Assistive Technology pointed me in the right direction for a funding grant and would continue to phone every now and then to see how I was getting along. Patty McDonald at the State Department of Aging got approval for the purchase of talking computer accessories for me. Mona Lee at the Department of Vocational Rehabilitation of our State Services for the Blind made it possible for me to receive a grant for professional editorial assistance on a regular basis, and Dan Tonge, from the same department, became my new computer tutor.

Before I could get approval for the computer accessories, I needed a faster computer, which my dear daughter bought for me. Thanks to all these people, I was able to set up a home office and to hire a two-person staff. Without this support the book could never have been produced. I am grateful for other donations that came from my brother John, my nephew Bob Comfort, my friend and neighbor Linda Berthy, and surprisingly, an author I have never met, Nancy Sorel of New York.

An old friend of mine, Carl (C.T.) Chew, generously offered to illustrate the work. Alice Volpe assisted in negotiating my way through the new world of book publishing, and it was J. A. Jance who introduced me to Alice. All the staff at Hunter House have shown patience and fortitude with me, and I appreciate this.

My colleagues Jan Quigley Park and Betty Hagman gave me useful professional advice. Others who read to me include Joan McClean, Laura Nelson, Alysandra Schwarz, Jennifer Carrell, Fleur Cowan, Alex Betzenheimer, Rachael Moore, and Christina Horst. Transportation, always a difficulty for those of us with vision loss, was provided by Linda Berthy, Kirstin Rogers, Lou Lambert, Myrtice Barr, and Phyllis Hansen. Among the people who have assisted in numerous other ways are Lauralee Carey, Carmen Blenman, Pam Jackson, and Judith Ryan.

In my search for personal stories for the book, I began contacting friends around the country, and they were a great resource both for the cameos and for clippings from periodicals and newspapers: Vincent Jolivet in Bothell, Washington; Johannes Laursen in Fort Myers, Florida; my brother John in Evergreen, Colorado; Ash Gerecht in Silver Spring, Maryland; Stella Sue Lee in La Jolla, California; Mary Lois Williams in Washington, D.C.; and Kay Shaw Nelson in Bethesda, Maryland; among others.

No other book of mine has demanded as much from me physically and emotionally, and certain people supported me here: my second family headed by Susan and Steven Carey and Susan's sister Ellen Oliver. These people, as well as Ruth Wilson, Linda Berthy, Tad Wolff, Kali Rose, my naturopathic doctor Bill Mitchell, and my primary care physician William ("Willie") Woo, believed in me and gave me the confidence to keep me going day after day, especially when the tension affected my vision. They kept reminding me of the contribution I was making to others with vision problems.

I want all of the above-mentioned people (and the others I may have left out) to understand how much I appreciate their support.

Foreword

As a physician who treats people with macular degeneration and other eye diseases, I see a great need for this book. I am aware of no other single source that provides the full scope of information needed by patients and their families. Betty Wason's book covers the nature of these conditions, ways to cope psychologically and in one's daily life, and the services and organizations that offer aid and inspiration.

I feel the special value of this book is that it comes from a person who is not a physician. Moreover, those most in need of reassurance and positive approaches to vision loss would be skeptical of hearing anything upbeat from an individual who has normal sight, and Betty actually has the disease. While I am ensuring that the scientific aspects are accurate and up-to-date, there is simply no substitute for the firsthand experience Betty brings to her discussion of vision loss and its many related effects on the individual and society.

As her ophthalmologist, I am honored to be treating Ms. Wason. My participation in this project is entirely voluntary. I have no financial interest in it, only a personal interest in seeing her produce this guide, which will be of benefit to so many others.

— **James J. McMillan, M.D.**

Important Note

The material in this book is intended to provide a review of resources and information related to macular degeneration and vision loss. Every effort has been made to provide accurate and dependable information. However, professionals in the field may have differing opinions and change is always taking place. Any of the treatments described herein should be undertaken only under the guidance of a licensed health care practitioner. The author, editors, and publishers cannot be held responsible for any error, omission, professional disagreement, outdated material, or adverse outcomes that derive from use of any of these treatments or information resources in this book, either in a program of self-care or under the care of a licensed practitioner.

Introduction

My own frightening experience with sudden vision loss inspired this book. I have been a professional writer throughout most of my 86 years, so my first instinct was to write about what it was like in a way that would help others.

But as the book grew from this first emotional reaction, I learned a lot about macular degeneration. I learned it is the chief cause of legal blindness, and what could and could not be done to help myself and the millions of others who suffer from the loss of vision it causes. I found suspected causes, and discovered why our advanced medical research scientists are still searching for answers as they poke around in the dim recesses of the human eye. I found out why no optical lenses have been perfected as a fix. What's more, I learned a great deal about macular degeneration's many low-vision cousins.

"Age-related" macular degeneration (AMD) was so named because it was noted mostly among older people. But it is now recognized that macular diseases strike every age group from toddlers to octogenarians. The most common form of hereditary macular degeneration, Stargardt disease, begins in childhood. According to my ophthalmologist, Dr. James McMillan, there are dozens of diseases affecting the macula alone, in addition to innumerable diseases of the retina, of which the macula is just one part. Although vision loss is the most-feared physical impairment among middle-aged and older Americans, knowledge about vision rehabilitation services is sorely lacking.

An important part of my research has consisted of personal contact with others who have various vision problems. After I was well into the book and conducting phone interviews with people in many parts of the United States, I came to see that all those with vision loss could benefit from the useful information I was collecting. Thus, this book is presented in such a way as to benefit anyone with impaired vision. For example, I visited low-vision clinics and support groups both for my own benefit and to learn more about the various services they offer.

Despite the common experiences of those of us with partial vision, I can state one thing unequivocally: every case of low vision is unique. While some people with age-related macular degeneration, Stargardt disease, macular dystrophy, diabetic retinopathy, and retinitis pigmentosa need magnifiers to read or cannot even read 20-point print, others can still drive their own cars and read the daily newspapers. Some people I interviewed for this book first experienced eye problems when they were just four years of age. The stories in these pages are of people who range in age from 30 to 90. Some play golf and jog daily. One woman skis and ice skates; another still manages to crochet and take the subway to work.

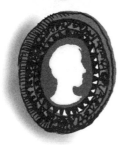

The stories are a fascinating portrait gallery of human beings determined to go on enjoying life regardless of severe handicap. I have been inspired by their courage, and I am sure you will be too. So this book, which began as a practical self-help guide for others who share my visual disability, has become a true-story book as well. "Cameo," as I use the term in this book, indicates one of these stories of someone who has a vision problem. The cameos are marked in the text with a symbol so you can find them quickly.

Today I can no longer read anything—not even my own handwriting—without a magnifier.

How then was I able to write this book? After I could no longer read my writing, I received a new Pentium computer equipped with JAWS and DECtalk accessories (Chapter 10 explores technology of use to those with low vision), enabling me to hear the words my touch-typing produced. I have not yet mastered this remarkable device, but it has helped with rough drafts of the book.

Most of this book was written in longhand, and transcribed to the computer by my remarkable and tireless assistants, Kali Rose and Tad Wolff. Their help was made possible by a grant from the Vocational Rehabilitation Department of the Washington State Services for the Blind. I am also indebted to innumerable friends who have given me volunteer help and their steadfast love.

I have persevered with determination and faith in the belief that this book would be of help to thousands of others struggling to adapt themselves to the harsh reality of vision loss. The interviews with people all over this land show the strength of the human spirit to be the greatest miracle of all. I now know that, if the first five senses are sight, hearing, touch, smell, and taste, the wondrous sixth sense is inner vision. Though I cannot read with my eyes, my mind and inner sight are clearer than ever.

A Special Message to Families and Friends

Upon hearing about my project, a social worker in a low-vision support group said to me, "I hope that in your book you will talk about the frequency of despondency among people with low vision—especially older women who live alone." The loss of vision in itself makes these women feel cut off from the world they used to know and this in turn makes them need a feeling of kinship with their families and close friends.

I hear people express these concerns frequently. "I have the feeling my relatives just don't understand what I am going through. They give me things I can't use—even books I can't read—and seem to think money makes up for the lack of companionship."

This complaint is understandable. I have suffered from it too, especially on important family holidays. "Talking books" make up for those we cannot read and vans take us places we can't drive to ourselves, but nothing takes the place of kinfolk who care. I have many wonderful friends and am grateful for all the nice things they do for me. But there are times, especially on holidays, when I long to be closer to those with whom I shared my earlier life.

If you are a relative or friend of someone with low vision, try to call the person at least once a week, if possible on a certain day and hour. This gives the person something to look forward to, makes her feel loved and remembered. If something comes up and you cannot make your weekly call, make up for it as soon as possible. One easy way is to keep on hand half a dozen blank greeting cards ready for your personal message. Of course, cards are welcome anytime.

When you are away from home, send postcards. If your friend is alone and cannot read your cards, she will save them until a reader is available. Of course, you can send e-mail if you have a computer, and there may also be a way to do this through your telephone service. The important thing is to let the visually impaired person know that she is remembered and is not alone.

Make a special effort to drop by as often as you can, if only to say hello and exchange hugs. Tell her where you are going, and ask if there is anything you can do for her.

A brief ride will be appreciated, perhaps to see some part of the town or city they are unfamiliar with, or to watch a beautiful sunset or a moonlit night. Having lost the ability to drive, people with low vision appreciate just getting into a car and going somewhere.

If you can't take your friend or relative to a restaurant, some fruit or a salad from the supermarket deli makes a nice surprise. A take-out meal from an ethnic restaurant is another good idea; an easy meal they don't have to prepare for themselves means a lot. Even those of us who used to cook and entertain friends find it difficult to do much in the kitchen when our vision begins to deteriorate.

If your friend or relative has a CD player, buy her a compact disc of her favorite music. Also, an extraordinary selection of audio books is now available, some humorous, some romantic, some deeply thoughtful. If she does not have a tape or CD player, you might present one as a gift. Tape players are quite inexpensive.

More important than anything else is the gesture, the mark of love that helps the person with vision loss feel she is a part of a caring world once more. You will be delighted by how this brightens her outlook on life, and most likely it will brighten yours too.

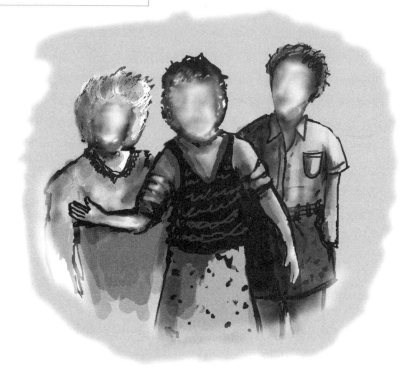

CHAPTER 1

How It Began for Me

I arrived early at the annual picnic of the Seattle Free Lances, my professional writers' club. It was the third Sunday of July 1996, a sparkling midsummer day. The spot was a delightful hilltop above a lake in a private park south of Seattle. I had been looking forward to this gathering of fellow writers and long-time friends. The group had a pavilion to itself and as other members came up the walk in a steady stream, I looked for people I knew. But while I could see bodies and attire distinctly, my friends had no faces. Not until they came within a foot or two of where I sat was I able to recognize them.

When the picnic was over and I was being driven home through downtown Seattle with its many skyscrapers, I had another shock. The buildings looked as if they were about to topple over. As I examined this phenomenon, building by building, I saw it was because the straight lines of the architecture seemed wavy and the blocks of stone and cement looked like misshapen lumps of clay. It was almost as if an earthquake had struck while I was at the picnic. It was a relief to get home. That evening, alone in my apartment and still shaken by the day's experiences, I thought back to what had brought me to this disturbing state.

It began in May with surgery to remove a cataract from my right eye. This was particularly important for me because three years earlier a mild stroke had damaged the retina of my left eye, leaving me with only peripheral vision in this eye. I had functioned all right with my one good eye, but the improvement offered by the cataract surgery would be welcome. Everyone I knew who had gone through cataract surgery had raved about how much better they could see within days of the procedure. My optometrist had been urging me to have an ophthalmologist perform the operation. It was a great shock when removal of the cataract made my vision worse rather than better.

On the day of surgery I was one of a half dozen women in the outpatient waiting room going through one preoperative step after another like large mannequins on a European town clock. The surgery itself was brief, and the next day, after the bandage was removed, my doctor barely glanced at my eye, exclaimed, "Perfect! Your vision is 20/40!" and departed. As I left I was handed instructions telling me to see my optometrist on the fifteenth and twenty-second of the month.

The First Frightening Weeks

The first weekend after the operation, I blithely drove around familiar streets without taking my driving glasses with me. But when I picked up the morning paper and could read only the headlines, I was bothered. I had always been able to read the smaller print. Then I attended a symphony concert, and after my eyes adjusted to the lights I saw all of the performers quite well, but every one had two heads. I joked about it afterward, but in reality I found the experience unnerving.

I didn't have time to dwell on the two-headed incident because I was in the midst of two writing projects, a mystery novel and a monthly newsletter. The pressure of deadlines was starting to catch up with me. My vision grew noticeably worse week by week. I had already arranged to discuss my novel with an agent and editors at a writers' conference in July, and wanted to have it ready by then. I still hoped that new glasses would correct my problem.

I was not permitted to see my ophthalmologist (the doctor who had removed the cataract) until six weeks had passed to allow the eye to adjust after surgery. When I told my optometrist, "I must have reading glasses, even if temporary ones," I was informed that my HMO had ruled that only the ophthalmologist could issue the prescription. I couldn't wait that long to resume my work—the few days' interruption I'd anticipated was already stretching into weeks—so I paid out-of-pocket to order glasses my optometrist thought would help. When they arrived ten days later, they were useless.

This was not an easy time. Evenings were unbearably long when I could not read, and the glare of the television screen hurt my eyes. I spent hours in the dim light of my living room listening to music and trying not to be fearful, filling legal pads with the final chapters of my novel in what proved to be an illegible scrawl. Days were difficult too; the only things I could do to occupy myself were gardening and taking long but careful walks.

Looking back, comparing my vision then with the way it is today, I would be more than satisfied to see as well again. But at that time, when my vision was deteriorating from one week to the next and no one was telling me why, I was angry and frightened. I grew so restless and distraught that I rarely got through a night without pacing my living room, imagining arguments with my doctors and optometrist. I developed what my family doctor diagnosed as "depression brought on by stress." I learned later that most everyone experiences these fears and uncertainties, but in those first few weeks there seemed to be no one I could turn to for answers and the anxiety was unbearable.

May turned into June, and when the all-important postoperative appointment with my ophthalmologist took place I was not in a forgiving mood. My doctor was a dour, humorless man I had never felt comfortable with. Whenever I had an appointment with him, an assistant (never the same person) would see me first. Then the doctor would enter, read the assistant's notes, mumble into his tape recorder, look at me over the tops of his spectacles, and, without comment, have me take the wall-chart test with its big letter E. I had been assured that he was a skilled eye surgeon, but I found him haughty and indifferent. My private name for him was Dr. Poobah, and I now focused my frustration on him.

"When am I going to get my new glasses?"

He gave me a surprised look and proceeded with the examination without answering. Finally, after he was finished with the eye chart and I thought he was ready to dismiss me, he came over to examine my eye more closely.

"There are two blood spots in your eye," he announced. "The retinist had better have a look. Make an appointment with him before you leave."

Having waited six weeks already I was not about to wait even one day more, so I stood my ground in the eye clinic and by 1:30 the retinist was able to work me in. The word "blood" had gotten his attention, and he ordered a fluorescein angiogram. I knew what this meant; I had had a fluorescein angiogram three years earlier when the stroke had damaged my left eye. In this procedure, red and yellow dyes are injected into a vein in the arm. The circulation of the dye through the blood vessels of the retina is viewed and photographed with a camera that can see all around inside the eye, revealing any abnormal substances there. Almost cheerfully, the technician said, "I hope we don't find more blood on your retina. That could be disastrous."

After the pictures were taken, I waited in the reception room for the prognosis. The technician came running out at close to five o'clock to assure me he saw no other blood but those two spots. I hurried back to Dr. Poobah's assistant to plead with her to have him send my optometrist a prescription for new glasses. "I need them now!" I cried. Then I went home, exhausted. It had been a long day.

I didn't know what "blood spots" meant. I was desperate to resume my normal life, and I still thought the right glasses would permit me to do so. No one had told me otherwise. A week after my checkup and seven weeks after the cataract surgery, I called the optometrist and found that Dr. Poobah had still not sent him the necessary prescription. My nerves snapped, and I sobbed for the entire afternoon.

The next morning my vision was much worse. When I tried to fill out some business forms downtown, strangers had to show me where to write the essential information and scribble my signature. I had trouble finding my way to the bus that would take me home. I was more frightened than ever.

I know now that stress could have brought on my partial

blindness. This incident in particular convinced me that stress influenced my vision, and by then—thanks in part to my unresponsive doctor and bad luck—I'd had seven weeks of stress in the extreme. By the time I got home, I was determined to find another eye doctor.

A New Doctor Gives My Affliction a Name

Even before the cataract surgery, friends and colleagues had told me I should have gone to the McIntyre Eye Clinic. Dr. David McIntyre was said to be the best eye specialist on the West Coast and one of the top five in the country. His clinic was some distance from where I lived, which posed a transportation problem, but frightened as I was by what was now happening to my sight, I decided I had to seek out the best possible care.

Dr. McIntyre originated a technique for cataract removal now in common use and had performed so many near miracles that his clientele included influential people from around the world. A slight, dapper man with a white goatee, his Old World manners matched the relaxed calm of his clinic—a marked contrast to the assembly line hustle of Dr. Poobah's clinic. When he heard my tale of woe, Dr. McIntyre tactfully said, "This sounds like a lack of communication." And after examining my eyes, he said simply, "You have macular degeneration."

I had no idea what macular degeneration was. I learned then that the macula is the central part of the retina, responsible for discerning fine detail. Typically, people with macular degeneration cannot see detail in the central part of their vision, although they retain their peripheral vision. The toppling skyscrapers I saw after my picnic outing in July are a common sign.

For a brief time, under the care of Dr. McIntyre's staff, my optimism rose sky-high. I liked the ophthalmologist assigned to me immensely. Harvard educated, James McMillan is tall and boyish with a quick smile. He makes his patients feel he really cares and has that most important of all qualities in a physician: he is a gifted listener.

I asked him point blank whether my vision loss was due to something that went wrong during the cataract surgery. He said, "I've looked for that but can see no evidence of it."

"Then what caused it?"

"I don't know. There's a lot about the eyes that still baffles the medical profession." This kind of honesty endeared him to me.

But my vision continued to worsen. When I wrote a long letter on my computer about everything I had gone through after my cataract surgery, I discovered I had to use a much larger type size than I'd needed only three weeks earlier for another project. Friends invited me to attend a performance of *Les Miserables* at a Seattle theater. When we entered the crowded foyer, my vision was so blurred that I couldn't see people clearly. The balcony seats provided a fine view, but when the house lights dimmed and the stage lights came up, all I could see of the stage was moving light and dark shapes. I couldn't fool myself anymore. My vision was not improving.

After successive optical lenses proved ineffective, Dr. McMillan ordered another fluorescein angiogram. When these pictures were examined, it was clear that my problem was wet macular degeneration: a buildup of abnormal blood vessels in the retina.

The experience in my right eye was typical of wet age-related macular degeneration. However, in some cases, wet AMD can develop slowly—it is possible that my macula had been deteriorating long before the doctor detected it. The two blood spots in June had apparently been symptoms that weren't taken seriously enough. Now Dr. McMillan said, "I've done as much as I can as an ophthalmologist. We need to bring in a retinist."

My choice was Dr. Jay Friedman, who had cared for me a few years before when the small stroke had damaged my left retina. He had acted swiftly, examined my eye thoroughly, and shown his concern by even opening his office for me on a Sunday. I felt it would be good to bring him into the discussion because he was familiar with what I had gone through before.

Dr. Friedman remembered me. Intense, brilliant, with a mind like quicksilver, he was willing to explain everything, but his descriptions of the eye's functions were often too complex for me to follow. He, too, took pictures, and, after seeing these, told me about a new method of treatment for wet macular degeneration: radiation. I didn't like the sound of that. I imagined losing my hair and taking on the gaunt look of cancer patients. I wanted a second opinion.

At my request, Dr. McMillan sent me to another retinist, Dr. David Drucker, who also took an angiogram (the fourth set of fluorescein angiograms!). At first he expressed doubts about the wisdom of undergoing this new and still experimental therapy. "I've heard about radiation, but, as I understand it, it has only been performed in three cities: Boston, New York, and Dallas. If you want to try this, you'd be better off going to Boston where doctors have performed it on other patients."

I phoned my daughter Ela, in eastern Washington, to tell her of my quandary. She called Drs. McMillan and Friedman and, from what they told her, felt the radiation was worth a try. "The radiation dosage is very low," she said, "no stronger than the x-rays we have all the time."

When I let Dr. Friedman know I had decided to go ahead with his proposal, I said, "I don't mind being a guinea pig as long as I'm not a sacrificial lamb."

"Hundreds of people have had the procedure," he tried to reassure me. However, I was to be the first patient in the Northwest to receive radiation therapy for macular degeneration. He produced a three-page consent form and, as he read it aloud, he repeated after nearly every paragraph, "We cannot guarantee anything."

At an earlier stage, I might have been alarmed, but by now I had made up my mind. I had to try to save what was left of my sight. I even hoped to recover what I had lost.

Trailblazing a New Treatment

When I went to the hospital, I thought I had been sent to the radiology department, but the sign over the entrance read "Swedish Hospital Tumor Institute." Surely this wasn't right. A tumor institute? Macular degeneration couldn't be a form of cancer, could it? Yet when I announced myself at the desk, the clerk said, "Oh, yes, Dr. Vermuellen is expecting you."

Sandra Vermuellen wore a tailored jacket above a miniskirt instead of the usual white doctor's coat, and she was slim and soft-spoken. As she explained the procedure, frequently referring to the pages before her, I tried to think back to what Dr. Friedman had told me. It had all gone a bit over my head because of the unfamiliar terminology. But now Dr. Vermuellen was talking about a series of radiation treatments and asking me to come in as soon as Monday for preliminary procedures.

Uneasily, I said, "I'd like to know a little bit more. After these treatments you are talking about, will I be able to read normally again?" By now I could not read at all. I desperately wanted the vision in my right eye restored.

But Dr. Vermuellen shook her head. "I'm afraid not. Dr. Friedman tells me you may never be able to read normally again."

No one had ever put it this bluntly before. Tears rushed into my eyes. "Never read normally again? Never?"

She came over from her desk to put a hand over mine. "I know it's a shock," she said softly, "but the treatments should prevent your vision from getting worse than it is now. And with help, you can adjust."

I went home deeply shaken. How could I possibly adjust to this? How could I live the rest of my life this way? I didn't yet know how unusual my case was. Many people with AMD go on reading for years, but the combination of the stroke damage in one eye and wet AMD in the other made that impossible for me.

Through yet another long night I prayed for help in making the right choice. Then a serendipitous string of signs reassured me. Over the next three days, I met three women named Kristin, Christina, and Chrissy. When I went to the hospital for a brain scan to prepare for the radiation series but could not read the elevator controls, a priest entered the elevator to show me which button to press. When I told the first nurse I met about these coincidences, I joked, "I guess that means Christ is on my side," but I was serious. I needed help, and I chose to take these signs as reassurance. That simple choice gave me the confidence I needed to proceed.

So it was that, on the day I returned to the tumor institute to have a radiation mask fitted, I was in a cheerful mood and feeling no qualms. To make the mask, which is worn during the treatment, a sheet of lacy white plastic was heated, then pressed tightly over my features, creating a visage nearly like my own. The doctor then marked on the mask the exact locations where the radiation would be administered. I asked the young attendant, "Have you prepared for this treatment before?"

"Oh, yes, lots of times," she told me. "But never for an eye treatment. You're a pioneer!"

"If I were a movie star, you could probably put this mask up for auction," I joked.

In a spirit of bravado, I later took the mask home, and in fact, I used it as part of a Halloween costume shortly afterward!

Dr. Friedman had said it would be three months after the last radiation treatment before I would notice any improvement. That meant another wait—this time until December.

Seattle Free Lances had its Christmas party in the home of the club's president. When friends drove me home, it was dusk and the lights of the city were glowing against a winter sky. We came to downtown Seattle and I almost held my breath, wondering what the skyscrapers would look like this time, remembering the awful sight of them twisted and toppling in July. But this time was a thrill—they were straight! I felt pure joy.

The radiation treatments did what they were supposed to do. They stopped the buildup of abnormal blood vessels within the retina. At my checkup at the end of December, Dr. Friedman was delighted to announce that he didn't see a trace of blood or fluid. So, I thought, "I've crossed the divide. Now things are going to be better."

This did not mean I could now read, but I had been warned of that. The radiation had at least arrested my descent into blindness and, it seemed to me, promised enough improvement to set my kite of optimism flying in the wind once more.

"What happens next?" I asked Dr. Friedman. He was elated that the treatment had worked. Other ophthalmologists in the region were already being alerted to radiation as an approved treatment for wet AMD.

"I can't predict how things will go in the future," he said. "I can only assure you that if the blood buildup had not been stopped, your vision would be a great deal worse. You and I are trailblazers."

I liked being a trailblazer better than being a pioneer. Pioneers are willing to travel in unknown territory; trailblazers leave markers to help others follow.

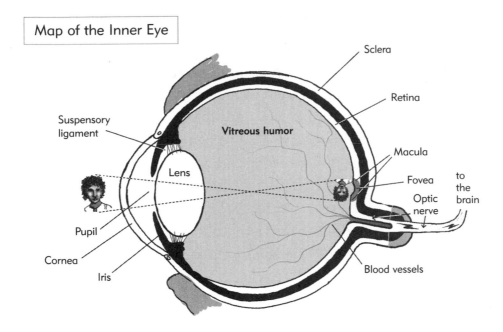

Map of the Inner Eye

Sclera

Retina

Suspensory ligament

Vitreous humor

Macula

Lens

Fovea

to the brain

Optic nerve

Pupil

Cornea

Iris

Blood vessels

CHAPTER 2

The Mystery of the Eyes

The eyes are the windows of the soul. Every emotion is expressed through them: a young lover's eyes glow with love, the eyes of an enemy may burn with hatred like hot coals, and a wink of the eye is like a secret understanding. When an old friend approaches, our eyes meet in greeting. Eyes often say as much as words, yet when we interpret other people's feelings and ideas by looking at their eyes, all we are seeing is the colorful iris. If the front of the eye can communicate so much, imagine how much more is happening behind the scenes.

The Structure of the Eye

The eye is something like a ball or a grape with a soft center—in medical textbooks, it's called a globe. The only part of this globe visible to the outer world is its window in front, the cornea.

The *cornea* is a transparent skin over the eye's outermost lens, which collects light into the eye. The cornea also covers the colored round *iris* and the iris's dark center, the *pupil*. What we see as the "white of the eye" is part of the outer skin called the *sclera,* which extends all around the globe of the eye. At the back of the eye is the *optic nerve,* the eye's direct contact with the brain.

In response to light, the pupil opens and closes to regulate the amount of light that reaches the inner eye. In bright sunlight or indoor glare, the pupil pulls tight like a purse string to compensate for the greater amount of light. At dusk or in a softly lit room, the pupil expands so that more light can stream in. The iris and pupil play the same role as the aperture in a camera, adjusting to the amount of light in the outer world—except in the eye it's all automatic.

Backstage at the inner eye

The real complexity begins backstage, with the inner eye. Fluid around the iris nourishes the eye's tissues. (Abnormally high pressure of this fluid causes *glaucoma*.) An inner lens rests just behind the iris in the front half of the eye. This lens permits the eye to focus on both close and distant objects. (If too many cells collect inside this interior lens, causing it to cloud over, this is known as a *cataract*.) Behind this internal lens is the soft center of the eye: a clear, jellylike substance called the *vitreous gel*.

Lining the entire inside of the eye is the light-sensitive *retina*. In most drawings of the eye, the retina looks like a thin line, but don't let that fool you. Inside the retina are millions of cells and a network of tiny nerves called *neurons* that relay images through the optic nerve at the back of the eye to the brain.

The retina is actually the innermost of four layers that cover the globe of the eye, each with a specific function.

The white fibrous outer layer, the sclera, forms a tough protective skin.

The next layer is the *choroid,* which contains hundreds of tiny blood vessels, the chief blood supply of the light-sensitive retinal cells.

Underneath the choroid is a thin layer of tissue called the *retinal pigment epithelium* (RPE), which has three important functions: first, to limit access of the blood of the choroid to the retina; second, to protect and help nourish the retinal cells; and third, to absorb light that the retina does not initially collect. This sharpens our daylight vision at the expense of our night vision and is why human eyes do not glow in the dark when hit by headlights like the eyes of cats and dogs do. The RPE absorbs excess light and prevents it from reflecting back out.

The fourth layer at the back of the eye contains the retina's neurons, which link the eye to the brain via the optic nerve. The retina consists of millions of cells, also called "photoreceptors" because they are light-sensitive. Of these, approximately 125 million are *rod cells* and 6 million are *cone cells.* The cones handle bright light, colors, and fine detail—especially in central (direct) vision. The rods are in charge when the light is softer, or dim, and play an important part in peripheral vision.

But there is still more to the retina. At the center of the retina, near the optic nerve, the *macula* reigns. The macula has its own rods and cones, but it has more cones than rods because the chief job of the macula is to clarify the small details in direct central vision. This tiny area of the macula—no larger than a typewritten letter "o"—is what allows us to read small print and street signs, sew fine stitches, and recognize the faces of our friends.

In the center of the macula is a depression, the *fovea centralis.* The fovea is composed entirely of cones, receiving the finest details striking the macula. An eagle has two foveae, both of which are more densely lined with cones than are the foveae of human eyes. This is what makes the eagle able to see a rabbit from a mile away, while a human being can see a rabbit from only a tenth of this distance.

Each part of the eye has an ongoing assignment and each takes orders from the retina, the boss of the back of the eye. The retina's continual contact with the brain means the "phone lines" are constantly in use and no "call waiting" is allowed. The iris and lens get their orders from the retina, the retina gets its orders from the brain, and all the neurons, muscles, rods, and cones get their orders from their respective managers—simultaneously.

Like roving TV cameras, the various muscles, cells, and nerves help to process the images brought in through the cornea to the vitreous gel. These images are then picked up and sorted out by the retina and sent on to the brain. The brain is the commander-in-chief of the entire body that makes multiple use of pictures and reports received from its many reporters and scouts—truly an awesome responsibility. Some of the pictures will be stored in the archives of memory for us to recognize later in dreams and storytelling. The only slowdown that occurs in this twenty-four-hour operation is in the dark, and even then the rods and cones are on constant call, remaining active even during sleep.

And that's not all! The same complex operation is taking place simultaneously in the other eye—coordinated by its respective part of the brain. Each eye has its own stimuli, its own pictures, and its own set of neurons, transmitted through its own rods and cones, macula, and fovea. To use a computer analogy, our eyes function as though they have the same motherboard. They work in unison from the same set of instructions from the brain. This tandem function is called *symbiosis*.

Not only are operations in the eyes going on in tandem, but as vision dims in one eye, the other eye will sometimes come to its aid. We may actually experience improved vision, at least temporarily. I observed this through self-examination at different times of day or night, holding a hand over one eye, then the other. I was astonished to observe how as one eye lost a degree of vision, the other grew stronger in compensation.

Macular Degeneration Affects All Age Groups

Over the centuries, vision loss, along with hearing loss and aching bones, has been considered an inevitable part of growing old. In the book of Genesis (27:1), Isaac is described as "old, and his eyes were dim"; because of this he couldn't recognize his own son.

Today, physicians consider macular degeneration to be the most widespread eye problem among older people in the Western Hemisphere. It is the leading cause of blindness in people over 50—more so than cataracts and glaucoma combined! And there is no cure. A September 1997 article in *Science* estimates that 11 million people in the United States suffer vision loss from AMD.

The proliferation of macular disease may in fact be attributable in large part to the much longer life span we enjoy today. Statistics show how the incidence of cases in the overall population increases with age. Nineteen percent of people ages 65 to 74 have macular degeneration, rising to 37% of the 75-and-older age group. However, macular degeneration does affect younger people—about 1.7 million people ages 45 to 65. These younger people are doubly impacted because they usually are still active in their careers. When author Stephen King was diagnosed with macular degeneration at age 49, the news sent a shiver among baby boomers everywhere.

Although the "A" in AMD stands for age-related, this term is now being called into question because more accurate diagnosis is revealing that diseases of the macula can strike in any decade of life, from 4 to 94. In addition, both Dr. McMillan and Ed Aleksandrovitch, director of the Macular Degeneration Foundation, have told me that "macular degeneration" is quickly becoming a generic term because there are so many diseases of the macula that can cause vision loss.

This new way of looking at macular degeneration was reflected in a symposium held by the American Association of Retired Persons in Washington, D.C., in April 1996. The discussion created a bombshell: a considerable number of research scientists expressed the belief that macular degeneration is caused by *disease*, that it is not merely degenerative, not just part of the aging process. If true, this changes many things. It suggests something can be done to halt the spread of the disease or at least reduce its impact. The results of that conference were reported in a full-page article in the *AARP Bulletin* of July-August 1996. The following October, when the annual national conference of ophthalmologists was held in Chicago, AMD was the key topic. In November and December 1996, the media picked up the trend, and after a dramatic presentation on the popular television news show "20/20" (a fitting name for a program about visual acuity), the tongue-twisting name "macular degeneration" was on its way to becoming a household word.

Two kinds of AMD

There are two quite different forms of macular degeneration: "wet" and "dry." In wet macular degeneration, also called subretinal neovascularization, new blood vessels grow abnormally ("neovascularization") and leak inside or under the retina ("subretinal"). Usually the blood has leaked from the choroid. When vessels or blood or even components of blood such as water, proteins, or fat get under the retina, they block the macula or disturb its cones. This is what makes straight lines look wavy and letters and numbers take on strange shapes. This problem affects about 20% of people with macular degeneration, but it can come on without warning and sudden deterioration can occur. This was true in my case—within two weeks of being informed that I had AMD, I saw a rapid decline in my vision.

Dry macular degeneration, also called atrophic macular degeneration, accounts for about 80% of AMD cases. ("Atrophic" refers to the death, or atrophy, of cells in the retinal pigment epithelium.) It develops more slowly than wet macular degeneration and may never become severe. The dry version is so-called primarily because there is no sign of fluid within the retina, simply a breakdown of cells and tissues in the macula. Dry macular degeneration differs so much from wet macular degeneration that a growing number of scientists believe that it is an entirely different disease.

Awareness of risk factors may help to prevent AMD, but there are very few fixes for either wet or dry macular degeneration (see Chapter 4). If caught in time, wet AMD can be stopped, and in some cases vision might even be improved with laser therapy or radiation treatment.

My Vision After Radiation Treatment

For me, radiation treatment halted the buildup of abnormal blood vessels and I noticed some improvement in my vision, although it didn't last. Several months after my radiation treatment, another problem arose. One day I noticed what I thought were pebbles lying on a tabletop. Then I saw pebbles everywhere. An hour later the pebbles turned into twigs, and by the next day the twigs had formed into a crosshatched pattern that looked like chicken wire. Wherever I looked, whether at a blank wall or a stretch of sidewalk, I saw chicken wire.

My ophthalmologist told me I was hallucinating—seeing things that were not really there. He said it was a common occurrence for people who had had eye surgery, and he predicted it would soon go away. But it has never gone away, so I have named it my "chicken-wire syndrome." It has now taken on an even stranger characteristic: often my field of view is covered by what looks like glittering fabric or a cloth of plaid design. Dr. McMillan has suggested that this phenomenon is a severe form of Charles Bonet syndrome, or phantom vision, in which the visual center of the brain "makes up" things to fill the void of information coming from the central retina. In any case, I take comfort in something else Dr. McMillan has said: "There are many things the medical profession still does not understand about how our eyes work."

• • •

Describing this chapter's tour of the inner eye was far from easy for me. To explore the mysteries of this extraordinary organism in understandable language required the help of patient and knowledgeable friends and neighbors. One was a premed student, Alysandra Schwartz, and another was Laura Nelson, who had recently graduated from college with a major in biology. Laura had a particular interest in my project because her mother, Katherine, who lives near Denver, has had a disease since her thirties called retinitis pigmentosa (RP) that is in effect the opposite of macular degeneration. In RP, central vision is unaffected, but peripheral vision deteriorates. Katherine's story inspired me to find out more about other vision problems. In the process, I came to learn that many of the services for people with macular degeneration are also offered to people with other vision diseases. (These services are discussed in detail in chapter 5.) I began calling friends in other parts of the country and was so fascinated by the stories people had to tell that I knew they had to be in the book. I call them "cameos," and you will find them at the end of every chapter.

CAMEOS

Katherine Nelson was diagnosed with retinitis pigmentosa (RP) in 1982, when she was in her thirties.

Doctors speculate that Katherine's eye disease is due to a recessive gene in her parents because none of her living relatives have the disease, but nothing else is known of the cause. "When I got older, I noticed my night vision was bad," she said. "Then, my peripheral vision went. I stopped driving six years ago, and now I can't see my whole face in the mirror or play Ping-Pong with my children—I can't follow the ball." Since RP affects both the rods and the cones of the retina, Katherine is losing her color vision too—she cannot tell the difference between blue and green or pink and yellow.

Despite deterioration of her vision, Katherine can still read and knit, "and I am very definitely thankful for that," she says. For Christmas, Katherine made her daughter Laura a latch-hook rug. She rides the bus all the time and is learning how to use a white cane. Katherine has kept her part-time job as an administrative assistant at a pregnancy crisis center. Her coworkers are very supportive and she appreciates feeling useful. She also sings in her church choir.

Katherine and her husband go to movies, and enjoy traveling around the country in their trailer. "He wants to take me to Chicago to the Foundation Fighting Blindness convention in the summer," she told me, "and I have yet to go see the color changes in the fall back East. But I'm especially fond of the ocean—we don't have much water in Colorado. You can't hear the mountains, but you *can* hear the water."

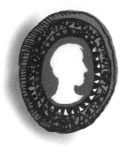

Although many people I interviewed for this book are in their seventies and eighties, I also talked with people who suffered vision loss while still young. **Alma Romero** was only 21 when she first noticed she was having trouble seeing. Her brother, **Sam Romero** experienced eye problems at the younger age of 13. They both have Stargardt disease, sometimes called juvenile macular degeneration, contradicting the notion that damage to the macula happens only as part of the aging process. Now 48, Alma first noticed a change in her eyesight during her first pregnancy when she couldn't pass a driving test. Determined not to let anything stop her, she obtained a special driving permit and searched for a doctor who would be helpful. Although it deteriorated suddenly, Alma's vision has been stable for 18 years now, and she continues to work full-time as a restaurant hostess.

Sam, also in his forties, put himself through college by working and with some help from Social Security. He edits an employee newsletter and alumni publication at California State University at San Bernardino, and does some freelance writing. He enjoys bowling, basketball, and dancing.

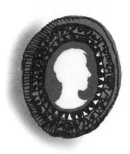

A few weeks before I sent this manuscript in, I had to revise, again, my perception of age in relation to macular degeneration. One evening I received a call from a telemarketer asking me to subscribe to the *Seattle Times*. "I would very much like to," I said, "but I have macular degeneration and can't read the newspaper." "That's funny," said the young man, "So do I!" It turned out that **Rob Hart** (this was his name) is now in his thirties, but has had dry macular degeneration since he was four years old. He has worked at the *Seattle Times* for two years, using special computer equipment to sell newspaper subscriptions over the telephone.

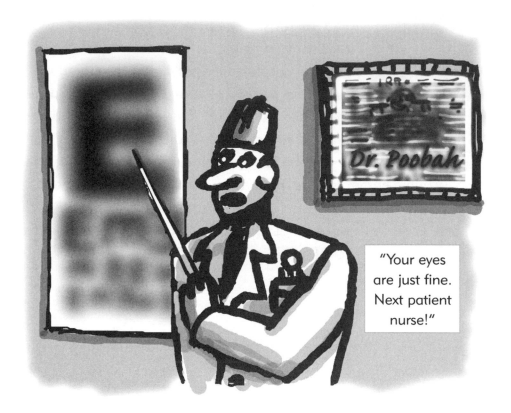

"Your eyes
are just fine.
Next patient
nurse!"

CHAPTER 3

About Eye Doctors

Despite all the extraordinary accomplishments in the medical field in the last half century, some American doctors seem to have acquired a bad reputation—almost as bad as the reputation of journalists. Is such censure justified?

In all professions certain practitioners are more skilled than others. I suspect we want sympathy for our unwell state quite as much as we want a quick cure—and this is what we don't always get from our doctors today. "Please, doctor, make me well again," is our inner plea. This is why the old-time family doctor who came into our homes was so beloved. With cheerful personal attention, the doctor felt our pulse and found a pill in his black bag that would probably help us feel better. The term "bedside manner" might seem out-of-date, but the old-fashioned doctor's concern may have helped us as much as those pills did. When the doctor told us we would be all right, we actually did feel better.

Different Kinds of Eye Specialists

In your search for proper, competent care, you will find several types of eye doctors. You are probably already familiar with *optometrists,* who attend four years of training at an optometry school. Optometrists measure the outer eye, the cornea, to determine what kind of optical lenses are needed to correct near-sightedness or far-sightedness. Optometrists give their prescriptions to *opticians,* who have had no medical training but understand the important technical skill of crafting lenses. Optometrists can also diagnose glaucoma and cataracts. Although they use the title "doctor," optometrists are not graduates of medical school and are not physicians.

The optometrist's role is an important one that fulfills the needs of most people with imperfect vision. But if you have an eye *disease,* an optometrist should refer you to a specialist such as an *ophthalmologist* or *retinist.* This is because optometrists' training does not permit them to diagnose conditions in the *inner* eye such as wet and dry macular degeneration. Although some optometrists specialize in low-vision problems, they will most likely suggest you see a specialist if you have any signs of trouble in your inner eye. Another reason to see a specialist is that they have access to a world network of all kinds of research. A specialist will be the first to know when possible new treatments become available.

Ophthalmologists are specialists who are graduates of medical school (physicians) and have continued for six more years in clinics and hospitals studying diseases of the eye. Ophthalmologists diagnose, research, and treat many of the diseases described in the previous chapter, including retinitis pigmentosa (RP), macular degeneration, and diabetic retinopathy. To see inside the eye, an ophthalmologist uses a special instrument called an *ophthalmoscope*.

Retinists have the same training as ophthalmologists and then go on for even more specialized study. Only a retinist can reattach a detached retina, for example. You will also need a retinist if you suffer from retinitis pigmentosa. While RP often strikes those in their twenties or thirties, it can happen to people of any age and, like macular degeneration, is incurable. In my case a retinist decided what treatment would be best to stop the buildup of abnormal blood cells in my right eye. This was a critical decision because the trouble spot was so near the fovea centralis.

If you are wondering which of these specialists to see, first discuss the matter with your family doctor or primary-care physician. Your family doctor will likely refer you to whatever specialist he or she thinks you need. However, if you are unhappy with this specialist, seek out another—and make sure whomever you choose is of the utmost competence. You also want your specialist to be familiar with the services that are available at low-vision clinics. He or she should be able to refer you to a clinic in your area.

The Importance of Empathy

In any doctor, the quality of empathy is as important as competence. You must feel comfortable with your doctor. You want a good listener who will pay attention to what you have to report on each visit, someone who will explain *empathetically* what has happened to you and what may happen in the future.

Always, and especially in the early stages, every patient fears blindness. If you feel you are just another number in your doctor's daily routine, you will leave the clinic in despair. But if your physician gives you reason to hope, to feel that life can still be good with pleasures yet to enjoy, you will not only be better able to face the world, but *your vision might actually be better.* Eyes are sensitive to and reflect one's emotions. Blood flows more freely to the brain when one feels happy and hopeful.

As I have spoken with people all over the country, I have been surprised by how often people have bitter feelings toward their doctors. People have told me that their doctors sometimes don't even answer their questions. So it is absolutely essential that your doctor have personal qualities that make you feel at home in his or her office. I referred earlier to a necessary "bedside manner." Feeling cared for is important, and you must find a doctor who is concerned with you as an individual.

The story of how I discovered I had macular degeneration is an illustration of the devastating effects of having a poor relationship with your doctor. I received conflicting information about what was happening to my eyes at a time when I was increasingly frustrated by my inability to see. My first ophthalmologist (Dr. Poobah) had an indifferent attitude that plunged me into despair and fear. As tension, fear, and worry can affect vision, I strongly feel this improper care hastened the deterioration of my sight.

Ironically, Dr. Poobah's clinic boasted of their "State-of-the-Art Technique Coupled with Old-Fashioned Care," but my new doctor, James McMillan, a specialist at Dr. David McIntyre's eye clinic, actually *has* these qualities. As I sat in Dr. McMillan's private consultation room waiting to see him for the first time, I overheard his conversation with an older couple. He had them laughing over some experience he recounted. I was impressed. Here was a doctor who cared for his patients in a truly old-fashioned way.

On a later occasion Dr. McMillan gave me laser treatment in my left eye (the one without macular degeneration) in an effort to clear up my "chicken-wire syndrome." I was not at all nervous when he directed the focused beam of light into my eye because I trusted that he cared about me. Being relaxed helped with this procedure; if I had been tense and had moved, the results could have been unfortunate. This is why Dr. McMillan is such a superior doctor—he makes his patients feel at ease, as does everyone at the McIntyre Eye Clinic. The pleasant atmosphere helps to ease patients' concerns.

People often ask why doctors aren't more honest with their patients. Doctors may reply that they are concerned with the patients' feelings and don't want to frighten them, but patients will be more frightened if they find they have not been told the whole truth about their condition. In some cases, a doctor might need to talk to a family member first who can then relay the information, giving the patient the feeling that the family is there and caring. But in most situations, doctors should talk directly with their patients, being tactful and honest, while at the same time reassuring the patients that others have adjusted to loss of vision and that they can too.

Many people state a preference for women doctors, perceiving them to be more sensitive and gentle. I do not think sensitivity is an exclusively female trait, although perhaps male specialists think the dignity of their profession would be undermined by too much "bedside manner." In any case, the role of the physician is that of healer, and this includes healing emotions as well as physical problems.

Humor is another valuable characteristic of a good doctor. Not that you should laugh at your affliction, but if your doctor can find any way to cheer you up, to help you out of the depth of your fear, that is indeed good medicine.

Being a Responsible Patient

Healing is not just the doctor's business; we must also do our part. Dr. McMillan has expressed to me his concern that many people with vision problems give up. They sit back and wait for the doctor to "do something," not realizing that most of what will improve their life is within their own control and will happen outside the doctor's office. He was particularly excited that I planned to include in this book stories of people who refused to stop living just because their vision had changed. I hope their example inspires you (as it has me) to make your own life full and rich.

When you visit your doctor, you can become a partner in healing by being an intelligent patient. Before your appointment, write a list of issues and questions to discuss with your doctor. Ask questions and make sure you understand the diagnosis and the procedures your doctor recommends. If you want to be sure you remember what your doctor says, take a tape recorder with you. You can listen to the tape at home or even share the information with your family.

Don't hesitate to report things that bother you. Such symptoms as blurring, night blindness, sensitivity to glare, severe itching, and sharp shooting pain might turn out to be significant. If your doctor dismisses any of these signs as unimportant, consider getting a second opinion. It is important to detect eye disease as early as possible.

Choosing a Good Eye Specialist

From both my own experience and talking with others, I have found that the best way to locate a good eye specialist is to ask around among people you know, starting with your family doctor. If your family and friends are not able to refer you to a good specialist, they may be able to ask among *their* friends. People who are pleased with their physicians like to recommend them. What's more, if you tell your ophthalmologist that five people referred you, he or she will certainly be happy—and it can only improve the connection you have with your new doctor!

Another way to find good physicians is to get references through an academy of ophthalmology or a local American Medical Association (AMA) chapter. If you are over 65, ask at your senior service center. Or try Seniors Helping Seniors, a nationwide organization that helps people plan how to pay for medical expenses. This is an independent nonprofit service, run by volunteers who themselves are seniors. Also ask people in your support group, professional club, or church or other house of worship.

Another consideration in choosing a doctor is the issue of transportation. If you are unable to drive, you will have to rely on some other form of transportation, such as friends or family, public transportation, or taxi scrip. (See Chapter 9 for more information about transportation.)

When choosing a doctor, pay attention to technical competence but also look for good communication skills. Your personal reaction—that gut feeling from deep inside—is important. Listen to what your mind and body are telling you about each specialist you talk to; this single choice can be critical to the health of your eyes.

Once you have a doctor you like, regular visits are important, and not only to check up on your particular ailment. Your specialist will be on the lookout for at least 20 diseases that result in low vision. Also, visiting your specialist even when there is no emergency is good because he or she might have more free time to convey new information about your condition. It is also an opportunity for you to share any new symptoms or developments.

If a doctor makes a small mistake or seems briefly unsympathetic, keep in mind that medicine is a demanding profession that requires practitioners to keep up with new research. Doctors must interact with all kinds of people and make difficult decisions that affect patients' lives forever. Let the physician know you appreciate her or his care. Doctors, after all, need understanding too.

Choosing Insurance Coverage

Sadly, financial considerations and your medical insurance might have much to do with your choice of doctors. When I was looking into how I would pay my doctor's bills with health insurance, I found that in the Seattle area there are as many as 40 insurance programs to choose from. It is impossible to cover all the options here because they vary depending on where you live and how old you are. People over 65 qualify for Medicare, which carries its own set of rules and limitations. (If you are approaching 65, you might want to check whether your current specialist accepts Medicare.) Also, various government programs exist for people with disabilities. Choosing the right medical coverage and, by extension, the right doctor, whose bills will be paid by that coverage, will take some work, regardless of your age and circumstance. You might want to ask for help from a relative or friend in researching medical coverage.

My own actions in this area might be an example of what not to do. In a panic over my failing vision and stung by my experience with Dr. Poobah, I was so concerned with finding a skilled and empathetic doctor that I acted in haste. True, I did find a wonderful doctor, but his office is more than 20 miles from my home and I have to depend on others for transportation. Also, the HMO that was covering my services from Dr. Poobah was the equivalent of Medigap insurance; that is, it covered the difference between what Medicare pays for certain services and what the doctor normally expects to receive. So in my first few months with Dr. McIntyre's clinic, I relied solely on Medicare. I did not anticipate a problem with this because my general health was good, but as it worked out, a minor illness landed me in the hospital and saddled me with an unexpected bill. In retrospect, I might have been better off had I done more research and found some additional insurance. Medigap would have covered most of that bill. Through the help of Seniors Helping Seniors, I later contracted with the American Association of Retired Persons (AARP) for Medigap coverage.

A checklist for choosing medical coverage

Here are some things to think about with respect to doctors when choosing medical coverage or an HMO:

- Are you restricted in which doctors you can see?

- Does this insurance provide coverage for alternative providers (e.g., acupuncturists, naturopaths)?

- What kind of referral process do you have to go through to see a specialist?

- Will you actually see the doctor when you have an appointment, or will you see an assistant?

- What is the typical caseload of a doctor covered by your plan? Will he or she be too busy to answer questions or address your concerns?

Also be sure the program you choose is not concerned more with "managed profits" than "managed care." So many complaints about managed care have been raised by unhappy patients to their representatives in Congress that changes in the system are already being discussed.

CAMEOS

Betty Burrill, 83, a retired geographer in Bethesda, Maryland, was diagnosed three years ago with pigment epithelium detachment, an incurable disease of the retina. After her diagnosis Betty found that most retinal specialists were reluctant to discuss the full implications of her disease. She wryly observes that this might be because a hysterical patient in the office is inconvenient. When she heard her diagnosis she didn't go to pieces, but inwardly she panicked because she had no close family to help her cope with her loss of sight. Her vision now is blurred to the point that she cannot read anything. She has since found several large support groups who meet at local hospitals.

Judy Schnitzer, who is in her early fifties, has had Stargardt disease for almost two decades. Judy lives in Encino, California, and serves on the board of directors of the Macular Degeneration Foundation, headquartered in San Jose. Judy has a master's degree in library science, has worked in real estate and sales and marketing, and more recently has volunteered in the nonprofit sector. Working with the Macular Degeneration Foundation has been very satisfying to her, because she feels she is helping others to see that life can still be good, despite macular degeneration. Along the way, Judy has collected a lot of very useful knowledge.

For example, Judy is the person who told me about the computer screen readers that are available for reading Web sites aloud and she, more than anyone I know, believes the need to educate eye specialists about low-vision clinics. Also, because of her own experience, Judy believes that people with macular degeneration can learn to read using their peripheral vision, by looking slightly above or below the text under a magnifier. "It is a bit tedious to learn," she says, "but it works."

Although her work has been rewarding, Judy says, "There are some days when I feel I've paid my dues for 19 years. I'm ready to see better." But then she always finds someone who has worse vision than she does and gets along well, and this inspires her all over again.

One of the people Judy noticed frequenting the macular degeneration list (see Resources) is **Tabby George**. Tabby lives in Austin, Texas, where she recently graduated from high school. She has written poetry and screenplays, was active on her school newspaper and the debate team, was involved in sports (swimming, track, and softball), and will soon be a student at Harvard University.

Tabby has had Stargardt disease since the fourth grade, but was misdiagnosed until her junior year of high school. Her optometrist found no refractive error in her eyes, so he told her parents she was lying about the blur because she wanted glasses. The blur in Tabby's vision grew steadily worse until she was legally blind. Finally, she went to Dr. Richard Lewis, a specialist in Stargardt disease who is credited with finding the gene connected to it. He was the one who determined that Tabby did in fact have Stargardt. Before attending Harvard, Tabby wants to travel in Europe for a year because she realizes that in four years she probably won't have the vision she has now. Tabby has overcome some common problems for people with low vision. To see her notes for the debate team, she used a thicker pen that doesn't bleed through the page. In restaurants she used her peripheral vision to read the menu. Her advice for other young people with low vision is "Don't be afraid to get involved in as many activities as you want. Don't lower your standards!"

Sign of trouble: when straight lines become wavy

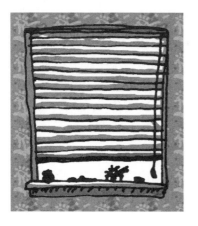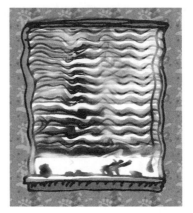

CHAPTER 4

Symptoms, Risk Factors, and Treatments

One of the first things to remember about any disease of the eye is that every case is different, even among people with the same disease. As I talk with other people who have macular degeneration, I am astonished at how different their experiences are from mine. I cannot read even large newspaper headlines, but a woman living across the hall in my apartment building is still reading her daily paper years after acquiring AMD. On the other hand, my color perception is in top shape—I still appreciate bright colors and can detect fine differences in color, yet another woman I talked with who has AMD has given up working in her garden because she cannot see subtleties of colors.

As you read the lists of symptoms and risk factors for the various eye diseases in this chapter, you may find some apply to you while others do not. In any case, see your eye specialist if you observe any of the listed symptoms or if any of the risk factors apply to you. These are warning signs of both common and rare eye diseases. It is always possible nothing is wrong with your eyes. But if there is, the sooner the diagnosis the better the chances that something can be done to save your vision.

Symptoms of Eye Disease

• **New glasses don't help.** If you get new prescription eyeglasses that make no improvement in your sight, consider seeing an ophthalmologist or a retinist. This failure of glasses to improve vision is the first and most obvious sign of an eye disease. It could indicate changes in your retina, not just in the lens of your eye. The fact that new glasses did not improve my vision after my cataract surgery was an important clue that something was wrong.

• **Blurred vision**. The first symptom I noticed was increased blurring in my eyes, especially when driving at night. If you are increasingly aware of blurs, notice where the blur is worst, testing one eye at a time. Is the blur spread all over? Do you feel like you are looking through a rain-drenched window? Is one side worse than the other? Is the blur in the center only? Out-of-doors, how far down the block can you see clearly? Where does the blurred area begin? Indoors, fix your gaze on specific objects and notice how much you can see of them, and whether the view is more complete if you move your eyes up, down, or to the sides. Where is the blurring thickest? Does your vision of a particular object vary according to the light? Many eye problems can cause blurring, including cataracts, macular degeneration, diabetic retinopathy (associated with diabetes, and the leading cause of blindness among working-age Americans), iritis (inflammation of the iris), and retinal detachment. To see if blurring is due to a problem in the interior of your eye, punch a tiny hole in a firm piece of paper with a pen point. Looking through this hole should make images clearer. If it does not, if you still see distortions and blurs, see your eye doctor.

• **Sensitivity to intense light and glare**. The second symptom I noticed was increased sensitivity to intense light. A consistent sensitivity to glare or light is likely caused by a cataract or possibly inflammation inside the eye, corneal injury, or "dry eyes" (dry eyes don't tear as much as healthy eyes).

• **Straight lines look wavy.** This indicates a serious change in your vision. Examine door frames, the lines of buildings (especially the horizontal lines of aluminum siding), and the slats of window blinds. Out-of-doors, notice overhead wiring, telephone poles, and skyscrapers. Also, see if letters and numbers are crooked. Your doctor may give you an Amsler grid, a fine-lined grid with a small black dot in the center. Make a dozen copies of this chart to keep around for testing. Cover one eye at a time, stare at the black dot and, without moving your gaze, see whether any of the grid lines are crooked. With a pencil or pen indicate on the grid where lines are wavy. If you do not notice any changes, date the test, then put it away and repeat the test in about a month. The doctor may want you to do it more frequently, but I found that if I did this test too often I could not observe any differences. If straight lines become wavy, tell your ophthalmologist right away because this could be a first sign of macular degeneration or another macular disease such as epiretinal membrane.

• **Double or distorted vision.** Cataracts, and sometimes diabetic retinopathy, can cause double or distorted vision. A few nights after my cataract surgery, I attended a symphony concert in which all the performers on the stage had two heads and the conductor had four arms. This has not happened to me since, but every now and then I notice a curious "jumping" or juxtaposition, like a double exposure with one picture on top of another.

• **Faded colors.** Eye disease often causes colors to fade or lose their luster. If you find that reds have become light pink or that you cannot tell the difference between indigo blue and forest green, report this change. Macular degeneration, cataracts, and hereditary retinal conditions can all cause problems with color perception. If other people often remark on the intensity or beauty of colors and you do not see them the same way, you should have your eyes checked.

• **Flashes of light.** Report any flashes of light, whether they are sudden and very sharp, or just a circle of flashing lights. Sudden light flashes can indicate a detached retina. A consistent sensitivity to glare or light is more likely caused by a cataract or possibly inflammation inside the eye, corneal injury, or "dry eyes."

• **Pain or pressure.** Pain and pressure can be signs of glaucoma, a condition in which the eye's fluid does not drain properly. If the discomfort is associated with light sensitivity, you might have a cataract. Pain might also be due to a bacterial infection. More generally, pain might be the result of eye strain, stress, or sinus disease.

• **Limited peripheral vision.** If your peripheral vision is closing in on you, yet you can read normally, you might have glaucoma. A limited periphery can also be a result of retinal detachment, stroke, or early retinitis pigmentosa.

• **A blind spot.** Blind spots can occur with macular degeneration, usually in the center of the eye. In retinal detachment, a dark shadow may appear, as though a curtain has been drawn across part of the field of vision.

• **Darkened or clouded vision.** If you have dimming or foggy vision, poor night vision, or are constantly needing a brighter light for reading, you likely have a cataract in one or both eyes. Vision can also become cloudy in diabetic retinopathy, and AMD sometimes causes a sense of fogginess.

• **Floaters, cobwebs, and smoke.** Floaters—dots or small circles that come and go—are caused by particles in the eye. This is different from "hallucinatory" images, which are created by the brain to fill a void where small parts of the retina are not working. If you see shapes that were not previously in your visual field, see your eye doctor immediately. Also report any change in the pattern of floaters to your doctor. The phenomena may indeed disappear in time, but you might even end up with my chicken-wire syndrome!

• **Itching.** It may be nothing serious, but itching can be a symptom of eye or eyelid disease including some kinds of infections. If it persists, report it to your eye doctor. Always be careful not to rub your eyes. To relieve itching, use eye drops recommended by an ophthalmologist.

You Can Help the Doctor

Even if you visit your eye doctor only once a year for an eye examination, you can check your vision yourself as often as you feel necessary. Remember, you are looking out from the inside, while your doctor is outside, peering in with an instrument. You may notice things about your eyes that he or she cannot see.

In general, check your eyes separately. Put a hand over one eye at a time and compare the vision of each eye. Look straight ahead for central vision, then look to one side, then the other, looking out through the corners, to the far left, the far right, down, then up, checking your peripheral vision. This exercise is something you should do regularly anyway to strengthen your eye muscles.

AMD, cataracts, and glaucoma are three principal causes of vision loss with aging. If you are getting on in years, treat seriously any symptoms of these three diseases that you notice. However, I have also listed some symptoms that I have been told might not necessarily be significant, because I feel that every curious or troubling visual peculiarity should be reported. *Some symptoms may simply be unknown because not enough people have reported them.* By making them known, we may be able to serve as researchers, in our own way.

For instance, for several years before I was diagnosed with macular degeneration, when I first awakened in the morning I would blink my eyes open and see a black disk that changed to white, then back to black again like a camera shutter opening and closing. When I opened my eyes wider, the disk disappeared. Much later I realized this black disk acted as a kind of weather vane for my vision. As my sight worsened in my right eye, the disk became larger and blacker. As my vision grew better after the radiation therapy, the disk shrunk and the edges grew fuzzy and irregular. Dr. McMillan thought this might be a normal blind spot in the center of the macula. Whatever the cause, if all of us report our symptoms for researchers to analyze, more warning signs will be known.

Also, retinal breaks may occur gradually and do not always cause symptoms. You might not know you have a disease for a long time unless your doctor happens to find it. Diabetic retinopathy may have no pain or symptoms at all, so people with diabetes should visit their eye doctors often.

Report any or all of the above symptoms to your eye specialist. They could be symptoms of other eye problems besides the ones mentioned. It is even possible to have wet AMD in one eye and dry AMD in the other, or a retinal break in one eye and cataracts in both. You will have a hard time noticing this yourself since a good eye will compensate for a bad eye, but your doctor will be able to detect the different diseases.

Diagnosis

Modern technology provides several devices that aid in the diagnosis of eye disease. *Ophthalmoscopes* are instruments that can look into the inner eye to get an overall view of the retina. *Ultrasound machines* use sound waves far above the range of hearing to map the shape of the eye. Sound waves are bounced off the surfaces of the eye and back into the machine, then converted into an image. *Slit lamps* are microscopes that illuminate and magnify structures inside the eye and are used with a magnifying contact lens.

Ann Elsner, an associate scientist at the Schepens Institute in Boston, has adapted the *scanning laser ophthalmoscope* (SLO) to see the deeper layers of the retina with infrared imaging. This type of imaging can even see through blood and cataract. The SLO enables earlier diagnosis of many retinal diseases that have traditionally been difficult to detect because they are in the back of the eye.

Dyes are also used in diagnosis, as in fluorescein angiograms (described in Chapter 1). This procedure entails an intravenous injection of dye that takes only a few seconds to reach the eye, and allows the doctor to see blood vessels more clearly.

Risk Factors

When September 1997 headlines reported a breakthrough in research on the causes of macular degeneration, hope leaped in the hearts of all those afflicted with this malady. Could this mean a miracle treatment, or a cure? But when the details were reported, the breakthrough seemed a letdown. The *New York Times* article reported a follow-up study to one of March 1997 in which researchers identified the gene that causes Stargardt's macular dystrophy, the most common form of juvenile macular degeneration. In September researchers announced that one in six people with AMD also had mutations in this gene, although in different parts of the gene. In the long run, the discovery of this gene is significant because it verifies that some forms of macular degeneration are hereditary and suggests that other eye diseases might be too. It may be that identifying this gene in young people could lead to counseling or treatment that could delay or even prevent the onset of macular degeneration.

Historically, macular degeneration has been thought of as a single disease that causes central vision loss, usually in individuals over age 65. This view is changing. Current thinking is that the disorder is a *group* of diseases that share a common result, affecting people of any age.

The following is a list of risk factors associated with macular degeneration and other eye diseases. A risk factor is a condition that increases the *probability* of getting a particular disease.

• **Eye disease in your family.** In the past several years, researchers have found genes associated with Stargardt disease, both wet and dry AMD, and retinitis pigmentosa. If several members of your extended family, including cousins, aunts, or uncles, are afflicted with eye disease, chances are great that you may be prone to it yourself. Also, because diabetes runs in families, diabetic retinopathy does too. Many eye diseases, including retinitis pigmentosa, familial exultative maculopathy, Sticker's syndrome, and stationary night blindness, have a genetic component.

• **Being female.** For some reason women are twice as likely as men to get macular degeneration.

• **Use of tobacco.** The use of cigarettes, pipes, cigars, and chewing tobacco increase your risk. One seven-year study reported in the Journal of the American Medical Association found that male participants who smoked more than a pack of cigarettes per day were two and a half times as likely to get macular degeneration as those who had never smoked. Another study showed that women smokers are at even greater risk than are men.

• **Caffeine and alcohol.** If consumed to excess, caffeine and alcohol are also risk factors for macular degeneration. The Mayo Clinic Health Letter recommends for eye health that men consume no more than six alcoholic drinks a week and women no more than three. Also, red wine contains antioxidant compounds (see Chapter 8) as evidenced by low incidence of heart disease in France in spite of a diet relatively high in fat, so red wine might be your beverage of choice for your allotted three or six drinks a week.

• **A diet high in cholesterol, fat, and sugar.** According to studies, such a diet can increase the risk of macular degeneration (and many other diseases too). Over time, animal fats may lead to clogged arteries that slow the blood flow to the brain and lead to blockage of the tiny blood vessels in the macula. The same low-cholesterol diet that is advised for those with heart disease and respiratory problems also reduces the risk of low vision. In addition, a lack of certain vitamins and minerals needed by the retina (vitamins A and B, zinc, and others) can contribute to several eye diseases. Likewise, a diet high in fiber, antioxidants, and natural foods is good for the eyes. (See Chapter 8 for greater detail.)

• **Exposure to ultraviolet (UV) rays.** Too much sun may play havoc with your vision. Studies have shown that UV rays increase the risk for both macular degeneration and cataracts. In one recent study, a 1% increase in UV exposure was seen to cause a 10% increased risk for cataracts. Those most at risk are Caucasian women, especially those of northern European ancestry with blue eyes. The effects of UV rays may result from too many hours of work in a garden or playing or watching outdoor sports. Exposure is lessened if one wears a brimmed hat and glasses with UV protection.

• **Other health factors.** There appears to be a link between diabetes and macular degeneration. People with a history of heart disease and stroke are also more at risk for AMD, as are those with other untreated general health problems such as hypertension.

When I read this list of risk factors, I shook my head in wonder. *Not one* of these possible causes applies to me. I have not touched a cigarette for at least 55 years. I don't care much for sunbathing, not enough to spend hours in the sun. I have spent a lot of time gardening in the spring and fall and have not always worn a hat. Could that alone have brought on my loss of reading vision? Dr. McMillan also considers heredity a significant factor, yet no one on either side of my family has had a serious eye problem. My blood pressure has always been normal. As a food writer I have always been conscious of proper diet—unknowingly following the very diet prescribed to avoid AMD. Although I had a ministroke in 1993, annual checkups since have always shown my arteries to be clear. So although it is always a good idea to be aware of the symptoms and risk factors associated with an eye disease, you might not exhibit any of them.

I would like to add two other possible risk factors that I have identified through my own experience and by talking to others. The first is *excessive exposure to glaring light,* such as that from a computer monitor or bright fluorescent lights. For a long time, if I spent more than half an hour before a computer screen, I would be temporarily blinded. Now my eyes are so sensitive to glare that I have had to stop using my computer monitor altogether. There is not enough scientific evidence for a causal link, yet my own eyes insist there is a connection. I did try using a glare- and radiation-reduction screen on the monitor, but it so dimmed the screen that I could no longer make out what was there.

Another possible risk factor is *cataract surgery.* This operation, in which the natural lens is removed because it has been clouded over time by normal production of cells, is an effective way to clear up clouded vision. However, my AMD was discovered right after cataract surgery, and I have now heard from other people who have lost vision when their cataracts were removed, so I feel I must mention this as a possibility.

For instance, the 80-year-old mother of my friend Patricia Hagerty found she could see almost nothing after cataract surgery. When her doctor wanted to remove the cataract from her other eye, her reaction was "No way!" My friend Dixie told me she knew of three people in Evergreen, Colorado, who were diagnosed with AMD right after cataract surgery. It also happened to Dr. Clare Buckland, 83, of Vancouver, British Columbia. Perhaps age has something to do with this phenomenon; perhaps the AMD was already present and simply became noticeable after the surgery.

When I asked Dr. McMillan about this, he attempted to find an answer through several channels, but none resulted in a definitive answer. He said, "We must often weigh several factors before making a decision. If removal of a cataract will make a great difference in vision and we can see no sign of other disease, we will recommend surgery."

Studies have concluded that if there is any incipient disease already in the eye, any surgery can exacerbate that condition. But even with today's equipment, it is not always possible to detect whether another disease is present, so doctors may perform surgery believing it is perfectly safe. This is an issue both doctor and patient must honestly consider when making the decision of whether or not to perform cataract surgery.

Treatments

Even if you have been careful to avoid risk factors and have had regular checkups with your ophthalmologist, you may still develop cataracts or AMD as I did. If this happens, your first question will be, "What can be done to help me?"

Nowadays cataracts are easily removed with surgery. Treatment of glaucoma is usually successful in people over 40 years of age. But until the 1970s, the answer to the question "What can be done about macular degeneration?" was "Not much." And for those with dry AMD, this is still the case. Doctors can only temporarily stop the downward spiral of dry AMD by recommending certain vitamins and minerals. Still, studies are underway in eye research laboratories all over the world to determine what causes eye diseases and what can be done to reverse their effects.

• **Laser treatments.** A laser is a device that generates an intense, concentrated beam of light. Laser treatment is usually administered in a specialist's office or in a hospital outpatient department. The doctor controls the laser by choosing its intensity, size, focus, color, and time of exposure. The heat from laser beams can be used to seal tears, stop bleeding, make tiny openings, and evaporate small amounts of tissue. For wet AMD, laser treatments are effective in stopping the growth of abnormal blood cells. In diabetic retinopathy, they seal blood vessels and dry up the fluids in the retina. In glaucoma, tiny openings in tissue are made to drain fluids, and a cataract can be helped with a laser by making an opening for light to show through.

If you receive laser treatment, you will be given eye drops to dilate the pupil and then some form of anesthetic. You will be seated in a dimly lit room where a doctor will place a contact lens on your eye. Depending on the type of anesthetic you are given, two methods can be used to focus the laser. One method is for you to look in different directions to expose the various areas of your retina. Another method is for a special mirrored contact lens to be placed over your eye to direct the laser. The procedure takes just a short time, but then you must rest with dark glasses for four or five hours or until the pupil returns to normal. Laser treatment does stop the blood vessel buildup in macular degeneration, at least for some time, but it must be repeated, depending on your condition. Laser treatment sometimes leaves a retinal scar, which causes a person to see a black dot in the center of one's gaze.

A 1998 article in *Parade* magazine reported a new use of laser treatment by Dr. Eugene de Juan of the Wilmer Eye Institute in Baltimore. Dr. McMillan says results of this treatment so far have shown that a majority of patients at least initially stabilize, with some improving and some regaining the ability to drive or read to varying degrees. It also apparently reduces the recurrence of unwanted blood vessels. Sometimes a treatment is initially promising, but later yields mixed results, such as the radiation treatments that I had. So I approach such reports with guarded—but real— optimism.

• **Radiation.** This treatment is still regarded as experimental by many ophthalmologists. For wet AMD, it is necessary to get radiation treatment as early as possible to halt the wild spreading of abnormal blood vessels. I received radiation treatment because the abnormal blood vessel growth was extensive as well as close to my central macula and made laser treatment too risky. (I describe my radiation treatment in Chapter 1.)

Immediately following this treatment and ever since, wherever I direct the pupil of my right eye, I see a circle of sparkling lights like a diamond broach with what looks like blue sky in its center. The sparkling lights do not interfere with my vision, but the patch of blue sky does. My retinist believes the results of radiation treatment were positive for me and had nothing to do with this "diamond broach." Consultations with other specialists have not produced any official answers as to its cause either. However, because it happened right after the radiation, and only in the eye that received radiation, I cannot help but think there is a relationship. So it goes with these still-experimental treatments to cure or halt loss of vision.

Very recently a slew of other possible treatments has been proposed, and some have been tested with varying results. In most of these tests, some patients showed improvement, some remained the same, and a few are worse off than before. All these efforts are still in the experimental stage, but science marches on.

• **RheoTherapy.** This treatment, also called plasmapheresis, "vacuums" the blood to remove toxic protein and waste material that hinder blood flow. The removal of this internal "sludge" increases capillary blood flow to the macula. The idea is to rejuvenate macular cells and thus improve vision. This treatment is expensive—requiring up to ten treatments costing as much as $2,200 each—and is not covered by Medicare.

• **Genetic treatment**. Now that a specific gene has been discovered in connection with macular degeneration and Stargardt disease, ophthalmologists can be on the lookout for early signs of these conditions in examinations and blood tests. People with this gene can take care to strengthen their immune systems with specific supplements or vitamins (see Chapter 8). Recently, retinitis pigmentosa has been found to have a genetic origin, and scientists have been working on a possible genetic treatment for RP in which the clone of a normal gene is inserted into a harmless virus that is then injected into the back of the eye. This might prevent or reverse the disease.

• **Retinal cell transplant**. Retinal pigment epithelium cells from fetuses and animals are being looked to as a possible treatment. In this most controversial of all the experimental treatments, cells from the eyes of a fetus would be transplanted into the eyes of a patient with macular degeneration. Scientists now know that animal cells can be harvested, grown in containers, and planted into a human eye. "Cells that are transplanted have the ability to interact normally with the other cell layers," said Dr. Marco Zabin, professor of ophthalmology at the University of California, San Francisco. "We don't want to raise false hope, but if the work keeps going as it currently is, we expect to perform cell transplants on humans in the next several years."

• **Retinal repositioning**. This operation involves cutting through the outer wall of the eye to the retina, which can then be detached and repositioned, moving the macula away from the leaking blood vessels. A laser is then used to kill the harmful tissue, without damaging the macula. In several cases, outcomes have been successful, but the physicians involved say the challenge is to make the procedure more predictable and to prevent complications.

• **PhotoPoint treatment.** In early clinical trials, one company (Miravant) has been able to stabilize and dramatically improve the vision of people with wet AMD. In the treatment, drugs are administered that have a special attraction to fast-growing tissue. Then, light is directed onto the macula to activate the drugs and regenerate cells. The results of the trial consisted of an improvement of up to four and a half lines on a standard eye chart for those who were treated at "therapeutic" doses of the substance. There are plans to move into the next stage of study to determine the long-term visual acuity of patients treated with PhotoPoint.

• **Strontium-90 treatment.** This is another experimental form of radiation treatment, which requires only one dose of this naturally radioactive metal, rather than several. In this treatment, a small piece of strontium-90 is actually inserted into the eye and held in place for a few seconds. As the radioactive substance decays, it destroys the nearby tissue.

• **BPD (benzoporphyrene) drug treatment.** QLT Phototherapeutics in Vancouver has been experimenting using their cancer drug, BPD, to alleviate the effects of macular degeneration. Used in combination with lasers, BPD clears out bleeding retinal vessels and slows further damage in new retinal blood vessels. At this writing, the drug is in final stages of clinical trials.

• **Antibody drug to vascular endothelial growth factor (VEGF).** Naturally occurring in the human body, VEGF triggers growth of new blood vessels. The antibody drug is designed to inhibit VEGF and halt progress of diseases caused by abnormal blood vessel growth, such as macular degeneration and diabetic retinopathy. This has had promising results in animal studies, with studies in humans due to begin soon.

- **Electronic retinal implants.** In this treatment, a tiny light-sensitive electronic chip would actually be inserted inside the damaged eye. (See Chapter 10 for a full explanation.)

- **Virtual retinal displays (VRDs).** A prototype VRD machine has already been built. With the VRD, an image is projected directly onto the working area of the patient's retina. (See Chapter 10 for more information.)

Other treatments for low-vision diseases are also being explored, though progress may seem slow because eye problems are complex and vary from person to person. Scientists are spending many hours in research laboratories searching for causes and cures. Research takes time and money, and treatments must be thoroughly tested before they can be publicly introduced. And people have fears about certain kinds of treatments. The use of thalidomide, for instance, sounds the alarm for those who remember babies born with distorted limbs because their mothers took this drug during pregnancy. Using radiation on the eyes, when it is normally used on cancerous tumors, might sound drastic. Another obstacle to finding cures for eye diseases is that some of these methods raise ethical questions. For example, transplanting cells from a fetus is unconscionable to some people.

Much is happening in eye research laboratories, and new findings are likely to be announced that will greatly change the picture. For instance, a drug that could destroy free radicals (substances in the body that can damage tissue) in the retina might be on the horizon. We are living in an exciting time. But because the problem of low-vision diseases is so vast, we need a range of solutions—not only $10,000 surgical treatments, but a $1.75 over-the-counter answer as well. Reducing risk factors is another approach, which, according to one expert, will drastically cut the numbers of people who develop eye problems later in life.

In the meantime, the best treatment will come from within each and every one of us. Most people get eye diseases in only one eye at first, and with one good eye a person can lead quite a normal life, as I experienced firsthand. It always helps, of course, to have faith and optimism, not to mention determination. If you want to go on enjoying life, remaining independent and proud, straighten up your shoulders, look on the bright side, and be grateful for the extraordinary abilities you have. A simple approach, but it works.

CAMEOS

In interviewing people for the cameos of this book, I asked each of them to describe their first experience with eye problems. Their answers were the equivalent of the list of symptoms in this chapter.

Norwegian by birth, **Gladys Nelson** was a by-line reporter for the *Seattle Times* for 20 years and has been a freelance magazine writer for ten years. We know each other from our writers' organization.

Gladys has always had her eyes checked regularly. Nevertheless, when she became aware that she could not see as well as she used to, she went to get new glasses. Her ophthalmologist gave her a copy of the Amsler grid so she could test her own vision periodically. When she took the test at home, she noticed a darkened area in one part of the grid. This proved to be the warning sign she needed. She made another appointment with her doctor and while she was in his office, he noticed hemorrhaging in her eye. He immediately canceled his remaining appointments and performed emergency laser surgery to stop the bleeding. The operation was successful. Her ophthalmologist also recommended that she take a food supplement called ICAPs that Gladys feels helped to improve her vision over the fifteen years she has been taking it. Gladys reads with the help of a handheld magnifier (8x). She makes use of large-print resources to keep up with what goes on in the world, and is still active in our writers' organization. In addition, she has recently started to take Norwegian language lessons!

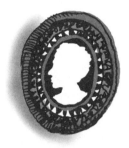

My editorial assistant, Tad Wolff, introduced me to **Dorothy Thorpe,** his grandmother. Dorothy, who is in her early seventies and lives in Spokane, Washington, couldn't figure out at first what was wrong with her eyes. Although she was working in an ophthalmologist's clinic at the time, she says her doctor was "one of the silent types" who, even though he diagnosed her with dry AMD, couldn't explain what it all meant. She finally switched to a woman ophthalmologist who proved altogether different: "She explained things so I understood them, and that made me feel good."

Despite her eye condition, Dorothy enjoys traveling to other countries, taking creative writing classes, and expanding her family tree with her knowledge of genealogy. She knows that heredity is a cause of macular degeneration, so she has been on the lookout for ancestors who had eye troubles. She recalls that her mother "was unhappy with her last pair of glasses. She couldn't put a finger on it, but she knew something was wrong with her eyes." Now it is known that when new prescription eyeglasses don't help, this can be a symptom of macular degeneration.

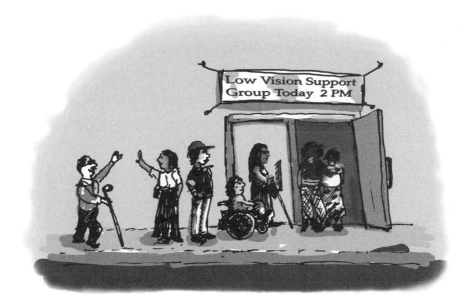

CHAPTER 5

A Vast Network of Services

Worse than hearing that I had an incurable disease—macular degeneration—was the discovery that even the latest prescription lenses from my ophthalmologist did not improve my sight. Surely a country leading the world in technological discoveries could produce eyeglasses that would compensate for diminished vision, whatever the cause. Yet when I looked through my new glasses, prescribed by an eye specialist at a clinic considered one of the best in the country, I could see no better than I did with no glasses at all.

It took me a while to accept this fact. One evening, with my new spectacles perched expectantly on my nose, I attended a summer

concert of chamber music, but even listening to a superb perfor-
mance by a cellist playing a rare instrument could not lift my spirits.
I could not read a word of the program notes, not even the heading.
My brand-new glasses were worthless.

After this discovery, I went to the drugstore and experimented
with nonprescription reading glasses. Although some of them
enlarged text to three times normal size, they only magnified the
problem: the blurs and the distortions were still there, only larger!
And my eyes hurt from straining to see through the glasses. I did
buy a circular magnifying glass that had a bubble at one side that
was a stronger magnifier than the rest of the lens, which I continued to use for a long time—particularly for reading prices in the
supermarket.

But before long I knew I needed something much stronger to be
able to read. I tried large-print books, but blurring still interfered
with my vision, no matter how large the print. The first two months
of my half-blind state were the worst, and it was during this time I
first heard about low-vision clinics.

Surprisingly, it was not from my doctors that I heard about
these services but from my brother in Colorado. Once I knew what
to ask for, some folks at a local senior center directed me to a low-
vision clinic in Seattle supported by a local charity, Community
Services for the Blind and Partially Sighted (CSBPS). With hope lifting my heart, I had a friend drive me there—only to be told my
name would be put on a waiting list, *if* I qualified. To qualify I had
to present a recent medical record proving my low visual acuity.
This I took care of immediately by calling my doctor and having him
send my records to CSBPS.

After an agonizing wait of several days, I phoned CSBPS to find
out if they could now help me. After a long pause the woman who
answered the phone verified that they had my records, and yes, I

did qualify for services, but it would probably be another four to six weeks before I would hear anything more.

Four to six weeks! In despair, I uttered a dismayed "Omigod!"

In a reproving voice, this unknown woman said, "We have a long waiting list. You're not the only one who needs help."

Low-Vision Clinics

Surprisingly, few eye doctors tell their patients about these organizations. Many doctors still dismiss patients with "Sorry, there's nothing more we can do for you beyond prescription eyeglasses." Doctors either do not know about the vast network of agencies and clinics that offer help to the visually impaired, or they just plain don't take the time to relay the information. The medical profession should be working more closely with the various organizations that provide these services.

Government organizations and independent charities are already working together through referrals and shared funding. If a state agency cannot provide a particular service, a caseworker may be able to tell you where to get help. Surprisingly, one does not have to be totally blind to get assistance from organizations that offer "services for the blind." Various organizations are beginning to use such descriptions as "partially sighted," "visually impaired," and "sight disabled," not only to make us feel better, but to let us know we can use their services even if we are not totally blind.

"Low vision" means you cannot see as well as those with "normal sight." What is normal? If you can pass a driver's test while wearing eyeglasses and can read printed signs without eyeglasses, your vision is "normal." Perfect sight is 20/20. If your visual acuity gets worse than 20/70, there may be cause for concern. The Social Security Administration's criteria for "legal blindness" is vision of

20/200 or worse in the better eye with the best optical correction. When eyeglasses do not improve your vision, you belong to the low-vision category and can take advantage of the vast network of support agencies. This makes sense, because when vision deteriorates to this level, typically one cannot drive a car and will have a hard time reading and doing other detailed work. Low vision is caused by macular degeneration (AMD and Stargardt disease), glaucoma, retinitis pigmentosa, and a dozen or so other eye diseases, so it is an extremely common condition.

The variety of services offered

Most services available through low-vision organizations are offered free of charge. If they are not free and you qualify for assistance, state agencies will often cover the cost. Here is a basic list of services and products available to you:

- Examination by a staff physician to determine which devices will be of most help to you, including magnifiers of all kinds to help in reading

- Courses in vocational rehabilitation for those who wish to enter or reenter the work force and thus remain independent

- Dormitories where out-of-towners can reside while taking independent-living courses

- Trained professionals who make house calls to help you make your living environment safer and more convenient

- Training with a variety of equipment such as fold-up walking sticks (very useful when crossing streets), talking calculators, watches, timers, and communication tools (such as large-print and talking books, and tape recorders)

- Volunteer help with bill paying, cooking, and transportation

- Emotional support or individual counseling to help you adjust to vision loss, as well as support groups that give you the opportunity to talk with others about similar problems and ways to cope

Many low-vision clinics also have a shop where you can buy devices to make your life safer, healthier, and more enjoyable. One of the most important tools available, and the best substitute for eyeglasses, is a powerful magnifier. Generally not available in drug stores, these powerful magnifiers can usually be purchased in low-vision clinics and through catalogs. The clinic's eye specialist will test you for many kinds of magnifiers: pocketbook size up to table-top size, with a vast range of magnification.

Closed-circuit televisions (CCTVs) are comparable in size to microfiche projectors, long used in libraries for magnifying films containing back issues of magazines and newspapers. I was so delighted with this device when I first acquired it that I named it my "Aladdin's lamp," after the manufacturer. When I place a sheet of paper under its lamp, a picture of the page appears on the CCTV's vertical screen, magnified as large as I like—up to 60 times normal size. The viewing format can be switched so that the background is either black with white characters or white with black characters, and it has a control for changing and fine-tuning the size of letters.

I can pencil changes on the printed sheet under the lamp of my CCTV. I can also read some postcards—those from people who have neat, concise writing. Personally, I find the glare of the screen hard on my eyes, but most people I have talked to don't have this problem and are very pleased with their CCTVs. These devices are available through low-vision clinics, catalogs, and sometimes ophthalmologists. Retailing at around $1,800, though, CCTVs cost considerably more than handheld magnifiers. The time comes, however, when price is no object. It is possible to find secondhand CCTVs—look in the newspaper or on bulletin boards at a Services for the Blind center. In time, the cost of new models may come down, too—or members of your family could pool money and buy it for you as a fine birthday gift. Recently some people who bought a CCTV on the advice of a low-vision specialist were able to receive funding from Medicare. If your doctor has suggested using a CCTV, you may want to file a Medicare "Part B" form to see if coverage is available.

Handheld and pocketbook magnifiers enlarge text to 8 times normal size and cost a lot less than CCTVs—generally $30 to $100. Some clinics may permit you to take home several kinds of the smaller magnifiers to try for a limited time. Magnifiers that do not require bulbs or batteries have been most helpful for my needs. Those with bulbs light up letters better, but one must be extra careful to turn off the switch frequently. A bulb left on overnight will be burned out by morning.

Finding and Attending a Low-Vision Clinic

Locating a low-vision clinic should not be difficult. Try the following:

- Look for "Services for the Blind" under the government listings in the telephone book, or have someone look this up for you. Ask if they know of a low-vision clinic in your area. Their operations may include such a clinic, but if not, they may be able to recommend one.

- Ask a member of a local Lions Club if the Lions know of or work with a low-vision clinic in your area.

- Inquire at a senior center, which can be a good source of information even if you are not yet a senior.

- Call Lighthouse, Inc. in New York City at 1-800-334-5497 for names of clinics in your area. Some areas of the country have their own "lighthouse" organization (not affiliated with Lighthouse, Inc.), so you should also check with your local directory assistance to see if there is a group of this name in your area offering services to people with impaired vision.

- Ask your ophthalmologist for a referral. If she or he does not know of a low-vision clinic and you eventually find one, be sure to pass on the information so your doctor can tell other patients about your discovery.

Once you contact a clinic to find out whether they can help you, the first step will be to fill out an application form. You must also request that your doctor's office mail or fax your medical records to the clinic so they will know your visual acuity and the nature of your vision problem. Some privately funded clinics require an "entrance fee" for admission and examination by their staff physicians. In addition, you will be expected to pay for magnifiers or other devices you want to take home with you.

If you have first registered at a state-supported Services for the Blind office, it is possible the agency will cover the cost of the low-vision exam, and in some cases the cost of devices needed. This depends on your financial circumstances, the seriousness of your visual disability, and your living arrangements. People with severe vision loss and limited financial resources can expect more aid than others who have better vision or greater resources. Likewise, people who live alone and have to pay readers can expect more aid.

After being accepted by a clinic, you will receive an eye examination from the clinic eye specialist that differs from what your ophthalmologist or retinist has done before. Because no two people with low vision have exactly the same problems or needs, this examination will be personalized. The physician will try to determine which of the available devices will help your particular circumstances. Sometimes magnifiers and other vision tools are sold in the stores associated with the clinic; if not, the clinic can refer you to special catalogs.

Dr. Irene Yang, the staff physician at my low-vision clinic, told me that people get more out of their visit if a friend or relative accompanies them. Your friend or relative can help you relate your story more accurately so the clinic staff can better understand what part of your vision needs improvement, and he or she will get a better sense of what you are going through.

The Seattle Lighthouse Project

One of the most thrilling experiences I had during the writing of this book was a tour of the Lighthouse project in Seattle. (The Seattle project is not legally affiliated with the national organization of the same name located in New York City.) One of the important services the Seattle Lighthouse provides is rehabilitation training. Here more than 300 people at a time, all of them with vision problems and many of them blind, are trained to enter or return to the workforce. Our tour guide, Ahna Miruhan, told me that contributors who support this amazing service include the Lions Club, the Boeing Company, and the federal government. Microsoft uses this facility to test new computer software that will be used by people with low vision.

It raised my spirits watching these people at work—all of them skillfully performing tasks that would have been impressive had they all had normal vision. One woman, blind since birth, was operating two braille computers at once. A man who had lost both eyes in an auto accident was testing new computer equipment, and he explained to us how the devices in front of him operated. One was a scanner on which he placed a magazine article to show us how it would read, in a synthesized voice that was easy to understand, down each column in succession. His sure movements and confidence belied his lack of sight.

In another room, a woman with macular degeneration was providing customer service with the aid of headphones, which channeled a phone line into one ear and her talking computer through the other ear. In the machine shop area, I saw a man working at his station, greatly absorbed in his project, checking a machine part stencil. He showed us a small magnifier that he had attached to his eyeglass frame that enabled him to adjust the magnification needed as he reviewed the details. He had found this device in one of the many low-vision catalogs.

Some of the people at the Lighthouse are employed by an offshoot company and produce such goods as rubber stamps, easels, and canteens that can be found in regular stores all over the country. The profits from these products help support the Lighthouse's programs. Wherever we went on the tour, the pride of accomplishment showed on everyone's face. It made me feel that anything was possible for people with diminished vision.

Operations at the State Services for the Blind

Another organization that provides valuable services to people with low vision in Washington state is the State Services for the Blind, with offices in seven cities. This agency proved the most helpful of all the low-vision resources for me; in fact this book could not have been written without them. (Check your local telephone directory for the equivalent group in your state). The services offered fall into three categories, according to the age of those who apply for assistance:

- Aid for children and their families.

- Training for seniors through an independent-living program. Today, many older people want to be active and continue to earn a living, or at least supplement their earnings.

- Vocational help for people who desire to return to the workforce through an agency called the Division of Vocational Rehabilitation. This is the most comprehensive program of all, with access to federal and state funds.

In some ways, Washington's State Services for the Blind provides similar training to that offered at the Lighthouse project. For instance, both programs offer training in computer technology. When I visited the Seattle office of the State Services for the Blind, I tried out several kinds of voice-activated computers. I learned enough to assist me in purchasing my own setup and I later enrolled in computer classes given by the Division of Vocational Rehabilitation.

I also attended a class in the State Service's home economics department to practice techniques in making household tasks easier, including kitchen chores (measuring, chopping, and much more) and sewing (threading a needle when you can't even see the thread!).

One of the most impressive services offered by the State Services for the Blind is the dormitory maintained for people who come to Seattle from out-of-town. Those qualified may stay at the dormitory with meals provided (free of charge) as they learn independent-living and working skills.

Home visits are also part of the services offered. I benefited from these when I asked if someone might come to my home to advise how I might improve lighting to avoid glare. I also received a talking calculator when I mentioned that balancing a checkbook was one of my headaches, and a timer for my kitchen with a loud alarm to warn me that I should return to the kitchen to prevent the soup from getting scorched. In chapters to follow I will describe in detail the techniques the fine people at these various agencies teach, and the devices sold by low-vision stores and catalogs.

Washington State Services for the Blind is funded by tax dollars from both federal and state budgets. Federal funds are also available to low-vision clinics to supplement their charitable collections. Our taxes help to pay for the equipment that makes such a great difference in the lives of people who have macular degeneration and other low-vision problems.

The Washington Talking Books and Braille Library

Of great assistance to people who can no longer read are "talking books," books read onto electronic media (tapes or CDs). On a recent visit to the remodeled and expanded Washington Talking Books and Braille Library (WTBBL), the first thing I noticed about the outside of the newly painted building was its striking sea-green color and its huge sign, declaring "WASHINGTON TALKING BOOKS AND BRAILLE LIBRARY." This special library is made possible through a program of the Library of Congress called the National Library Services for the Blind and Visually Handicapped, with 57 branches around the country. Inside I found walls painted a bright coral that contrasted with the green plastic of more than 170,000 volumes on cassette, in braille, or in large print. More than 380 volunteers donate their time every year, repairing tape players and receiving and checking tapes and players.

The Seattle branch of the Talking Books Library serves about 11,000 people annually, with a circulation of almost 500,000 books a year. The National Library Service funds the books, cassettes, and tape players; private donations pay for large-print books; the Washington state legislature provides the operation moneys for WTBBL; and the Seattle Public Library administers the accounting and the printing. There is no charge to the blind, visually impaired, or physically disabled to use these services.

WTBBL provides other valuable services, too. They sponsor a book discussion group attended by both sighted and unsighted people that meets once a month. They demonstrate and loan out CCTVs for people to test before purchasing. In addition, they provide on-site book reading and taping services, specializing in Northwest authors and topics not likely to be carried by the national catalog of low-vision books. Most people place orders over the telephone or by e-mail. WTBBL ships out books by mail, prepaid, and borrowers can return them by prepaid mail.

This library even has a special children's room. This room keeps lots of "normal" books with braille added directly on top of the printed words so blind and sighted readers can share their reading enjoyment (a mother, for example, will read the words while guiding her child's fingers over the braille). The room also holds books with other tactile stimuli such as protruding "cookie monsters" and plastic sculptures of lions and giraffes. Some books have a button to push that tells the book's story out loud; researchers have found that sound is very important to children's development. Until I visited this library, I had not been aware of how many thousands of children are either born with low vision or acquire it at an early age. WTBBL is giving these kids an important start in life by introducing them to books they can feel and hear. (See Resources for information on how to contact a Talking Books Library in your state.)

The Legacy of Helen Keller

Some agencies for helping those with low or no vision are government supported, some are supported by private charities, and some are service organizations. These agencies are found in all 50 states, as well as in Canada, Great Britain, and many other countries. In the United States alone, at least a half dozen national organizations raise funds for research and maintain facilities for people with low visual acuity.

The story behind this network of philanthropic nonprofit services goes back to Helen Keller. Most people know about Helen Keller and her wonderful teacher, Annie Sullivan—how this blind and deaf child learned to speak and proved to have a brilliant mind and charming personality. She graduated cum laude from Radcliffe College, mastered foreign languages, and wrote several books.

In 1925, the now-famous Helen Keller gave a speech before a gathering of men in a philanthropic organization formed only eight years earlier, the Lions Club. At the end of her lecture, Helen urged the men in her audience to "Go forth as knights of the blind in a crusade against darkness." They took her challenge to heart, and vision problems became the primary focus of what became the International Lions Club. Though the Lions Club is one of the youngest major service organizations, it is now the world's largest, with 1.4 million members in more than 180 countries. Through its Sight First program, the Lions Club helps people with serious vision problems. One of the services of this program is maintaining an eye bank for people in need of corneal transplants.

Many charities have been inspired by women like Helen Keller. The Seattle Lighthouse operation, for example, grew out of a small women's group that banded together in the 1920s to do charitable work. But the tradition of helping people with eye problems goes back even farther in the history of the United States. In fact, it was 53 years after the signing of the Declaration of Independence that the country's first public effort was made in training and educating people with vision problems. By the end of the nineteenth century, all but a few states had established schools for blind people. The New York Free

Circulating Library for the Blind opened in 1896, and its 1,649-volume collection of braille books and 492 pieces of music became part of the New York Public Library in 1903. In 1904, Congress allowed books for blind people to be mailed free of charge through the U.S. Postal System, and federal moneys were first made available for vocational rehabilitation through the Smith-Hughes Act of 1917.

Ironically, it was in the depths of the Great Depression that the Randolph-Shepard Act of 1936 paved the way for states to open offices offering services for the blind with national funding. Other strides took place during the prosperity following World War II, when annual funding for federal and state rehabilitation programs (for disabled people including people with low vision) more than quadrupled to over $150 million from 1954 to 1965. Every five years the Randolph-Shepard Act is amended to address the changing needs of people with disabilities. In addition, recently the Americans with Disabilities Act has mandated that employers make reasonable accommodations for disabled people. This may make it possible for those of us with vision loss to reenter the marketplace.

The good news about vision loss (if we can bring ourselves to think about it this way) is that more is done to help people with low vision than with any other single affliction. What's more, people in the past didn't have nearly as many organizations and resources as are available today. Help for people with vision loss clearly had small beginnings, but it has evolved into a network that extends all over the United States and many other countries.

CAMEOS

One thing I noticed in my dealings with various agencies serving people of low vision is that many of the people working in them have low vision themselves. Their help and encouragement have been all the more effective because they truly understand the frustrations and despair that accompany loss of vision.

Mona Lee, 59, a counselor with the Washington State Services for the Blind, has partial sight, but full optimism. She was the caseworker assigned to me when I first asked for help from the organization. With Mona's help I was able to qualify for services through her department, including the help of readers and drivers, as well as training in the kitchen. In addition, Mona took me seriously when I explained I wanted vocational rehabilitation (at age 85!) rather than just the opportunity to learn independent-living skills. She helped me get a grant for vocational rehabilitation that made writing this book possible. She and her husband enjoy riding their tandem bicycle and do some backpacking as well. In 1998 they completed a 1,046-mile bicycle tour from Boston to Toronto.

Elise Matthews, 42, is a field supervisor for a Washington State Services for the Blind office that covers all of Snohomish County. She has had at least five eye afflictions since childhood, including glaucoma, a scarred retina, cataracts, uveitis (inflammation of certain parts of the eye), and iritis. All of these problems stemmed from juvenile rheumatoid arthritis, which affects the immune system. At one point in her life, Elise's knees functioned so badly from the arthritis that she had to wear leg braces.

Elise had such a hard time with her handicaps that she considered suicide. "I was too much of a chicken about it—I did not want to live. I had to physically start going through the motions, then my heart caught up with me. What got me started was getting involved in something just for the sake of getting out." Elise then decided to learn to snow and water ski, and in turn these accomplishments gave her the confidence and motivation she needed to go on in life, and "even to interview for a job."

Elise has held many jobs since then. She coordinated recreational activities for Washington state and was instrumental in getting the local public television station to produce descriptive audio services for people with low vision. Elise says she is grateful for the opportunities she has received through state funding, including her education. Her current position with State Services for the Blind gives her tremendous satisfaction. "My job gives me purpose. It means a lot to be giving something back, helping others."

Because she is no longer able to drive, her employer provides her transportation. Elise carries her delightful smile wherever she goes. In the future, she hopes to do as much global travel as she can. "It's fun—it's the perfect freedom."

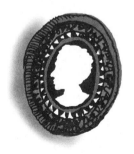

Seventy-eight-year-old **Audrey Ruud,** of Burien, Washington, ignored the signs of AMD, thinking it was nothing more than dirty glasses or the stress of caring for her seriously ill husband. Within days of her husband's death, doctors confirmed her near-total vision loss. Audrey admits she was initially angry and discouraged. But at Community Services for the Blind and Partially Sighted, she learned practical and emotional skills to continue living. Now she leads an area support group for people with low vision. Audrey says, "I wasn't happy about losing my sight, but I see now that there was a reason. These people needed someone to help show them how to keep on living." Audrey has organized shopping expeditions, boat tours, library trips, and a night out at a dinner theater. She's a living example of how rich life can be even with vision loss.

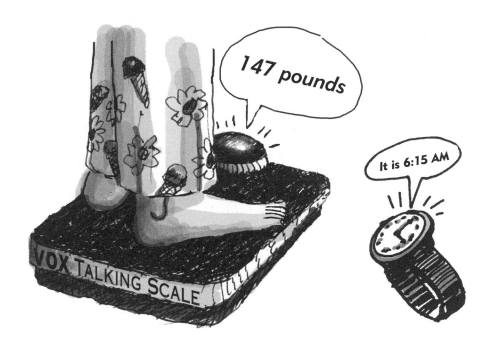

CHAPTER 6

Making Your Home Life Easier and Safer

After I registered with a low-vision clinic, four members of the staff appeared at my home in succession. These helpers not only offered suggestions for better lighting, but one came equipped with a roll of white Velcro and a pair of scissors and pasted little white markers everywhere. She was hard at work for a good hour making clear targets of thermostat controls, radio dials, and certain temperature settings on the stove and microwave. That was nearly two years ago, and the white tabs are still in place serving me faithfully.

Then, when I was accepted by the vocational rehabilitation section of the State Services for the Blind, a woman from the staff came to my home on two separate occasions to see what she could do for me. She was cheerful and empathetic, and urged me to call her with any problems I had. She supplied the support and help that the old-fashioned family doctor used to be noted for.

Many of the suggestions that follow come from tips I received on such visits. Others have been gleaned from people I have talked with, and some are from low-vision catalogs (see Resources for a list of these catalogs).

Floors and Lighting

Because of diminished vision, we are often unable to see potential dangers right under our noses. An experienced professional will realize which areas of our homes are potentially hazardous and can suggest inexpensive ways to eliminate the risks of stumbling or burning or cutting ourselves.

Slippery floors where carpeting leaves off pose a hazard for people with low vision. Shiny hardwood floors are pretty to look at, but may lead to tripping or falling. Small area rugs can be truly dangerous. Tape down the edges of floor coverings and place nonskid material underneath area rugs.

If you have macular degeneration, you may find you don't need lights on during the night, except for a tiny nightlight near the baseboard. This is because the retinal rods used in peripheral vision also help you to see well in dim light. In fact, I find that when I have to get up at night, it hurts my eyes if I turn on an overhead light. A good alternative is *diffused* light set up to penetrate corners and the parts of the rooms where you must walk. A light that remains on all night in a bathroom or hall should prove particularly useful for illuminating door sills and dipping floor levels.

Be sure you have good lighting in halls and inside closets, and make light switches easy to turn on. If switches are not located next to the door or entry of a room, consider getting lights that are controlled by touch or by motion detection.

Walls and ceilings should be painted white to increase light reflection and to show up darker pieces of furniture by contrast.

Steps are always hazardous if not well lit or marked, and they should have handrails. If possible, mark the edges of steps with white—perhaps by a strip of muslin sewn onto carpeting or a strip of Velcro applied at the edge. It might also be useful to carry around a pocket flashlight to throw light in front of steps.

In the interests of both comfort and safety, it may be that one of your helpful visitors from a low-vision agency can suggest a better and safer arrangement of furniture so you have a safe path even in dim light. Anything with sharp edges that you could hurt yourself on, like a footstool or hall table, should be in a well-lit spot that is not in your line of travel.

If you have macular degeneration and are among the lucky ones who can still read, your table lights should probably be shaded. Gooseneck or other adjustable lamps can be focused at different widths at a particular spot on a page. Some of these lights also incorporate magnifiers. For those who wish to do detail work like knitting or writing by hand, such lamps can make an enormous difference. Even some people who thought they could no longer read have been pleasantly surprised after trying the right muted or focused lighting.

In the Living Room

Be sure your sofa and chairs are a comfortable fit for your body. Comfortable seating will improve your eyesight by increasing the flow of blood throughout your body. But don't forget about other people when arranging furniture. When friends come to visit, you will want them to linger and chat.

Lighting in the living room is of particular importance. Dimmer switches for your primary ceiling lights can help you adapt to light changes. Halogen bulbs, available in hardware stores, are best for bright light that is glare-free. But take care that halogen lamps do not tip over, and that no flammable materials (such as synthetic fabrics and old papers) get close to the bulbs; the heat they give out is so intense they can cause fires.

For people with 20/20 vision, a day of clear skies and bright sunlight is welcome and having sunlight pour into the family room is a joy. But for me and others with macular degeneration, bright light can be torture. It hurts my eyes—everything I see seems to be covered in a gold cloth. I am blinded by it and must wear sun shields, sometimes even indoors.

In my east-facing office, I had blinds of a soft deep blue installed. When closed tight they are like curtains—they shut out the morning light and soften the room. At midday when the sun has shifted to the southern sky, I can pull up the shades and enjoy clear light without glare.

As you live with vision loss, your sense of touch will become more valuable to you. In the vast spaces of living rooms, feel each piece of furniture as you pass through. Develop your sense of touch and you will be identifying almost everything without the use of your eyes. Fabric textures will help you identify your clothing. The rough edge of a quarter, the smooth edge of a nickel, and the size of a dime will give away the identity of a coin very quickly, as will the characteristic edges of your house keys. (In many countries, different denominations of bills are different sizes. Though this is not true of U.S. paper currency, instruments that identify paper bills are available from low-vision catalogs.)

In the Kitchen

Many aspects of cooking can be more difficult if you have low vision. Take-out food can be your caterer when company comes for dinner. Potlucks are also a good idea—your friends can help with the cooking! You will need to cook sometimes, though, and there are many ways to make this an easier and safer experience.

Accidental fires are a perpetual hazard in kitchens: skillet fires can happen by accident when you have turned on the wrong burner and a stray piece of paper or plastic or the wooden handle of a kitchen tool catches fire. *Keep a box of baking soda handy,* always in the same place near the stove, with the top open. Toss baking soda onto the fire to snuff it out. I have found that most fire extinguishers are difficult to operate, even by people with total vision, but keep a small one in the kitchen at all times.

When you can't see perfectly, it is much easier to get burned when cooking or from something that is hot. Likewise with dishwashing: if you can't see where you are setting down a glass, it may fall onto the floor and you will have broken glass everywhere.

Remember to shut cabinets and drawers right away to avoid bumping your head or hip on a sharp edge.

Knives are another potential danger in the kitchen. Keep them stored in compartments or on magnetic holders. When you need sliced foods, either have the market slice them for you, or try a Magna Wonder Knife from the hardware store. These knives have a slicing guide that adjusts thickness to help you when cutting loaves of bread and bricks of cheese.

Have a first-aid kit handy in case of cuts or burns.

In my days as a cookbook author, I planned kitchens. I became familiar with labor- and time-saving principles when I was a home economics student at Purdue University. Organizing shelves, I knew, was important—canned fruit on one shelf, soups on another. One should also put the most-used utensils, plates, and cups where they will be easy to reach. If you live alone and have very few dishes, as I do, put only a small number of dishes in the inside front of cabinets so you do not need to poke around in the back, feeling your way to the right piece. A "lazy Susan," or turntable, will help you reach things easily. I keep a couple of skillets hanging from hooks on the wall and the most-often-used bowls and saucepans in the closest lower cabinets. In short, make sure your favorite tools are accessible.

In the kitchen, diffused lighting works best. Long fluorescent lights can be installed beneath the upper cabinets, illuminating the countertops but not shining in your face.

When measuring liquids, the first rule is to use light-colored containers for dark liquids (such as soy sauce or red wine vinegar) and dark-colored containers for light liquids (milk or orange juice). Use nested measuring cups (those that provide a separate cup for each measure gradation, i.e., 1/4 cup, 1/2 cup, etc.) instead of relying on your dim eyesight to gauge the amount of liquid in a glass measuring cup. Some of these cups are metal with a long flat handle. One way to distinguish which cup is which is to punch (with a nail—you can get someone to help you with this) a series of holes in the handles. For instance, use one hole for 1 cup and four holes for 1/4 cup.

A simple way to determine whether a glass is full is to sink your finger down inside to feel how far the liquid comes up. (Be careful, though, the liquid might be hot.) Your finger can also be a simple temperature gauge. You can identify leftover foods in the refrigerator by touch as well, especially such foods as grapes, muffins, or chicken.

As a visiting social worker showed me, marking items in the kitchen can help with both safety and efficiency. Follow these simple tips:

- Stick small squares, triangles, and rectangles of white Velcro on dials to indicate where to set the temperature for the oven and the time on the microwave. On the microwave, a triangle could point to the start button and a square could indicate the stop button.

- Velcro or felt stick-ons can also help you identify what is inside cans or jars, as can labeling them with a bold, black marker.

- To identify frozen foods, use colored ties to close up bags of vegetables, fruit, or leftovers.

- Easily identify the contents of packages by writing in large letters on big, bright labels and placing them on the box or can.

I have found tricks like these especially helpful at night when the room lighting is dim.

In the Bathroom

Next to kitchens, more accidents happen in bathrooms than in any other room of the home. To help make your bathroom a safer place, follow these guidelines:

- Have some kind of no-slip bottom on your bathtub. Rubber mats and stick-on designs are available at hardware stores.

- To avoid slipping on wet bathroom floors, always have a rug (with a rubber backing) or a bath mat at the ready to soak up water.

- Have railings installed along the walls of the tub and the shower to help guard against slips.

- Test bath or shower water with your hand before getting in to make sure it is not too hot. If you have control over your own water heater, you might want to have someone check the thermostat to make sure it is set at 120 degrees. This setting is recommended by Washington state law to reduce the risk of scalding and to save energy.

- Make sure your bathroom has good, bright lighting with an easy-to-reach switch to help prevent stumbling or tripping.

- To help you read the labels on medicine bottles or boxes, keep a small magnifier in the medicine chest or a vanity drawer. You could also buy self-stick blank labels at an office supply store and print the names and dosages of medications on them in large black letters. Even better, to identify certain important medicines by touch, wrap them with rubber bands or Velcro.

The Glow of White

When I was an art student many years ago, my teacher explained that white light is the combination of all colors and black is the absence of color. White is brighter than any single color—which is why the white highlights on my canvas glowed from across the room. This phenomenon is partly due to the bright quality of white itself and partly to contrast: placing a white object against a dark color like black or deep blue makes the white seem even brighter.

White is important as a beacon in the dark; notice at night how much better you can see white cars or people dressed in white.

This principle explains why white Velcro is so useful for identifying places on dials and why white walls show up the contours of a room. The only color that can compare with the visibility of white is "Day-Glo" red. Office supply stores sell paper stickers in various colors of Day-Glo, and I have used these to mark such items as computer and stereo controls and my favorite pens. Day-Glo yellow and light yellow-green also show up well, but blues, especially light blue, tend to disappear in the dark. Surprisingly, dark reds can appear to be black to those with dim sight. These color differences are important to keep in mind when you mark things in your home.

Out of the House

Special care is also needed when you are visiting in someone else's home. Some modern homes have rooms on several levels and for anyone with limited vision, steps between levels can be booby traps. If you find yourself in such a situation, ask for an escort to lead you through the unfamiliar territory—both going and coming.

When you visit restaurants, theaters, and cafes where lighting tends to be dim, pay attention to the ground where you walk and the lighting overhead. Hallways often have changing levels—hold someone's hand and maybe even take along a small flashlight to light up the path to your seat. In a restaurant, you can ask the host for a table where the glare of lights won't hurt your eyes. Your flashlight can also help you see your food.

A Place for Everything

Everyone knows the frustration of misplacing things and muttering to oneself, "Now where did I put those keys? My glasses? The pen with the best point? That letter from Betsy?" But when one's sight is fading, this experience is worse because you must *feel* your way around, touching tabletops and lifting cushions, peering through the blur.

I can still hear my mother's voice, "A place for everything and everything in its place." But I *do* try to follow this maxim because not being able to find things like scissors or keys is maddening. So I figure out a good place for frequently needed items and *try, try* always to put them there after I use them. It has taken me some time to get in the habit, but I am determined. Here are some of my rules:

- *House keys:* I put them in the same spot whenever I come home—inside the pocket of my purse as soon as I walk through the front door.

- *Wallet:* I keep my wallet in my purse with the house keys and remove it only if I change purses.

- *Eyeglasses and sun shields:* Although eyeglasses don't make much difference to my vision, my eyes feel more protected when I wear them. I keep these and three wraparound sun shields in a convenient bowl in the front room. (I have three colors of sun shields that I use depending on the light.) When I spot a pair out of place, I immediately return them to the bowl.

- *Address book:* Mine is a loose-leaf book with alphabetical dividers. I would be cut off from the world if something happened to it, so I always keep it next to the phone in the living room.

Telephone Tips

Making phone calls remains for me the greatest daily headache. Primarily this is because of all those numbers: dialing one for long distance, area codes, sub-area codes, and extension numbers. Another phone phenomenon is that irritating computerized voice that says "If you have a touch-tone phone please press 1 now," followed by a long series of options, "For customer service press 1 . . . for billing press 2. . . ."

If you find all this pressing depressing, there is a way around it. Most systems are set up to connect rotary telephone (the old-fashioned dial telephone) users with a live person because they can only interpret signals from touch-tone telephones. If you don't press 1 and just wait on the line, someone will answer your call.

I own two phones with very large number pads and a choice of "quick buttons," which are supposed to make it easier to dial repeated numbers, but because I can't see well, I have trouble remembering which quick button will dial whom. As I mentioned above, I keep my address book by the telephone at all times. Mine has loose-leaf pages so I can write numbers in big, bold strokes and not worry about wasting space. I can buy extra pages so it is easy to add and subtract names.

Some people prefer a Rolodex-type address system because its cards are spacious enough to accommodate large, bold numbers with notations at the bottom as required. You can hold these cards close for easier reading while you dial. They can also be thrown away and replaced. A further advantage of a Rolodex system is that it can be kept right next to the phone, solving the issue of having to hunt around the house for a stray scrap of paper on which to write.

Magnifiers Come in All Sizes

In the early stages of vision loss, you may find that inexpensive magnifiers in a drugstore or optical shop work for you. Some people find that even store-bought eyeglasses will help for a time, but not even the strongest eyeglasses helped me—they only magnified the blurs and distortions.

Instead, for two dollars I purchased a five-inch glass bar magnifier in an optical shop that turned out to be very useful in the first months of my vision loss. These magnifiers are intended to help in reading telephone names and numbers in fine print, but I used that little bar for a good six months for many things, from names on envelopes to instructions on food products.

You may need training in how to use magnifying devices properly. Many people grow frustrated because they don't know the correct distance at which to use them, which varies depending on the type of magnifier. The staff at your low-vision clinic should be able to help you.

Just as useful as that straight glass bar was a round magnifying lens with a small bubble at one side and a handle, also purchased at a drugstore. The bubble enlarged letters more than the rest of the glass. I used the device at the supermarket to read prices and signs in large print, though it did not help at all with normal reading tasks.

When these little pocketbook devices were no longer strong enough for me, I found what I needed at a low-vision clinic. My favorite magnifying device is called a "stand magnifier" or a "standing cone." A lens about 2 inches in diameter is supported in a frame with legs so it sits about 2 inches above what you want to magnify. Standing cone magnifiers are inexpensive—only $30 versus $80 for a magnifier with a light bulb—so I bought three: one for the telephone table, a second for my desk, and a third for the living room. Another reason I have three is that the frame is an inconspicuous black, and I am apt to misplace them several times a day. (I am currently experimenting with attaching Day-Glo stickers around the legs so I can spot them more easily.) At any rate, I always know each room has at least one magnifier.

In general, I do not like any of the devices that require bulbs and batteries because if you fail to turn off the switch, the bulbs and batteries burn out. New bulbs are not only costly, but you can buy them only at a low-vision clinic. The most effective and least expensive light bulb magnifiers are those with halogen bulbs. These bulbs cost $8 to $9 apiece, while ordinary incandescent bulbs are a bit more expensive at about $12. The batteries for these magnifiers can be bought at some hardware stores, but make sure you get the right size. The easiest way to buy bulbs and batteries is to take the device with you and try them out in the store.

Another solution to the problem of batteries is a magnifier with a plug-in cord. However, not only are you limited to where you can use this magnifier (only where there is an outlet or as far as an extension cord can reach), but the cord itself can be a safety hazard waiting to trip you. Other magnifiers are available, including no-hands, strap-to-your-head binoculars that can be used for watching television. There are also closed-circuit televisions (CCTVs), the tabletop magnifiers mentioned in Chapter 5.

Most low-vision clinics will permit you to take home one or more of their appliances, including CCTVs, to try out and discover for yourself which kind suits you best. This is a great help because so many kinds of magnifiers are available. As time goes on, it may be that your favorite handheld magnifiers are no longer strong enough and you will need to return to the clinic for an exam to try some with greater magnification. Though we hate to think of it, for many of us our vision will continue to deteriorate, making it necessary to switch to magnifiers of greater strength—just as eyeglasses need to be renewed from time to time.

Your Walking Stick or Cane

It is vital that you get out-of-doors every day for fresh air and exercise, and a daily walk should be part of your schedule. White canes or fold-up walking sticks in white with a red stripe can be acquired through a low-vision clinic or a catalog. Mine, which is white with a red stripe near the point, was a gift from a caseworker from a low-vision clinic. When I unfold this stick and hold it in front of me as I walk, it has quite an amazing effect on traffic. Cars immediately slow down. Drivers can see that white cane even better than they see the person holding it. The advantage of the fold-up kind is that you can carry it in a tote bag should a friend or neighbor drive you to a park for your daily walk.

A lesson in the best way to use a walking stick is helpful. With the walking stick fully extended, you can use it to gauge whether the sidewalk is sloping or the pavement is uneven. Most important, though, it is a signal to let others know you are visually impaired. This can help in crossing streets—it will display to drivers that you have low vision. It can also be a way of letting people know your low-vision status when entering buildings or visiting shops.

Don't be ashamed of your vision! Remind yourself how many other people share your problem, and use your walking stick as a red and white badge of courage.

Other Helpful Devices

A growing number of other products are both a source of amusement and a big help to people with vision problems. Many of these products are available through low-vision catalogs. Here are some of the ones I own:

- Talking calculators make it easier to balance your checkbook. Mine gets used every month.

- Heavy-lined checks with plenty of spaces and templates to help you write in the correct spaces make check writing easier.

- Talking wristwatches announce the time at the push of a button. I like my talking watch. The female voice is crisp and businesslike.

- Clocks and calendars printed in large numbers allow you to see the time and date at a glance.

- Big, bold timers help make cooking easier. Mine is hung on the wall so I don't have to look around, wondering where I put it down last.

Here are a few other products available in the catalogs:

- Glow-in-the-dark door handles that make it easy to negotiate your way in the middle of the night.

- Round mirrors that enlarge your reflection.

- Every large-print game you could imagine: Scrabble, Monopoly, playing cards, cribbage, backgammon, and more.

- Easy-threading and automatic-threading needles that make the toughest part of needlework easier.

- Talking thermostats, microwave ovens, caller ID units, money identifiers, compasses, scales, toys, and dictionaries with large print.

Many of the magnifiers, walking canes, and other things mentioned in this chapter can be ordered from special catalogs such as the Lighthouse, LS&S Group, and Maxi-Aids. (See Resources for ordering information.) If you see something in a catalog that sounds intriguing, call your low-vision clinic and ask if they have the item in stock. If they do, drop in and try it out for yourself before buying. Unfortunately, often what appears to be just what you need in a catalog may not be right in your particular situation.

These products are intended to make your life easier—less

stressful. If they don't make your life easier after you have learned to use them properly, you may need something different. Because your everyday life will be very different now, you will also need some personal skills for reducing the frustrations that will inevitably confront you. Some techniques for reducing this stress are described in the next chapter.

CAMEOS

Here are some of the ways others have found to make their home lives better:

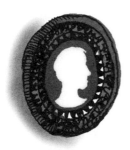

Thom Ingebretson, 71, from Modesto, California, was diagnosed with macular degeneration when he was 66. He explains how to navigate with impaired vision: "You have to study contrast. Having no depth perception makes a difference when you're stepping off a curb or going down stairs. Many people use the same carpeting on their stairs as they do on their floors because it looks better. All of a sudden you're stumbling down stairs you didn't know were there. After a while, you look for things—like handrails." Thom takes his cues from his environment. "I'll often walk behind people so I can notice when they step up or down. I mimic what they do. There are a lot of clues around if you look for them."

Anne Thompson, 72, of La Jolla, California, loves to cook. However, since she developed glaucoma in 1990, she can no longer read recipes. To make life easier, Anne has begun a new project with the help of her two teenage granddaughters. Using her CCTV, Anne reads each of her favorite recipes into a tape recorder. This well-organized collection of recorded recipes will be useful to Anne, should she continue to lose her sight. Anne hopes to make her "talking recipe book" available to the public as well. She teaches literature at the Braille Institute once a week and says, "One of the advantages of working at the institute is that it gives me an anchor so that if my eyesight gets worse, I'll have the support I need." When her husband is away for the day and she has to cook for herself, Anne creates one of her favorite easy-to-prepare recipes: an upside-down pancake, with pears or apples, accompanied by a glass of non-alcoholic wine. "I just create a party for myself," Anne says with a laugh.

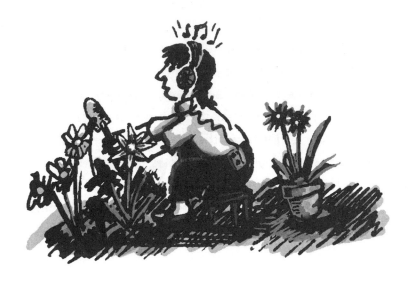

CHAPTER 7

Dealing with Stress

In our fast-moving world, everyone experiences stress at some time or other. But for those of us who have lost vision, stress is a much more continuous affair. Wasted time spent feeling over tabletops for misplaced house keys, days spent searching frantically in closets or dresser drawers for some article of clothing—these frustrating times pile up until the accumulated stress makes a person want to scream, or weep!

Stress and People with Vision Loss

To find out more about how stress affects people with vision loss, I visited noted Seattle M.D., psychiatrist, and Jungian analyst Ladson

Hinton. Dr. Hinton is a tall man with a gentle manner and a soft laugh. We were seated in his small comfortable office, which looked out over a spreading tree. I started by asking him what he would say to a person with a vision problem who had come to him for help. His reply startled me. "Before I would give any advice, I would want to know as much as possible about this person. Each individual is different and there is no one right course of action."

He went on to say that some people have experienced heavy losses in their lives before, so eventually they are able to come to terms with the stress from eyesight loss. Others find it extremely difficult to adapt. Among those who struggle most with loss of vision are people like hard-driving business professionals, who are accustomed to being in control of themselves and others. Another type are those who have been avid readers all of their lives and are at a loss when they cannot turn to favorite reading material. A third type are people who have never had a serious loss before and feel unjustly punished. "But," Dr. Hinton added, "I have also known people who for years and years had a whole lot of stress but never developed any illness."

Dr. Hinton explained why vision is so important to us. "We see the world with our eyes. When we cannot see clearly, it is like being cut off from life. Our language expresses this. We say, 'Seeing is believing,' and we speak of the eye of God and the evil eye."

At the time I spoke with Dr. Hinton, I felt sure I was one of those adaptable people, given all the ups and downs I had experienced in my life. However, a couple of days later as I was trying in vain to use my computer, I found myself distraught and furious with life because I had no control: my vision loss meant I could no longer do things that previously had been easy.

Those of us with even partial vision loss experience this loss of control. Muscles tighten every time we must peer through a magnifier, trying to make out a phone number. We copy the information in bold writing and struggle to see while dialing, only to receive that robotic voice: "The number you have dialed is no longer in service." We want to scream every time we need our house keys and stumble around peering through the haze, touching everything on tabletops where they might lie, trying to remember where they were "put away."

There are times when I feel like Sisyphus, the man in the Greek myth who was condemned to roll a heavy rock up a steep hill into an abyss. Whenever he approached his goal, the stone rolled back down the hill and he had to start over.

I felt like Sisyphus following my "pioneering" radiation treatment. At first I saw definite improvement in my vision, but then the chicken-wire syndrome—a pattern of wire netting covering most of my field of vision—made its appearance. Dr. McMillan tried removing the eight-year-old cataract from my left eye, thinking this might clear up the chicken wire. For about a week the wire did grow faint, but then I was struck by a rare virus, which settled in my eyes, the most vulnerable part of my system. The chicken wire came back in full force and my eyes were as bad as before. At that point, I felt like crying and feared I would soon be totally blind. But the virus ran its course and soon I was in control again.

My experience is typical of this cycle of stress: your vision worsens temporarily, and fear creeps in like a shadow. Your constant worrying begins to drag you down. Your uneasy mind makes small events in the real world seem like demons out to punish you, and you feel powerless. You are far from powerless, but stress has magnified small irritants into threatening enemies.

When I am happy, I want to do things and I have extra energy. When I am upset, I tire quickly from performing everyday tasks. A number of people have told me how exhausted they have become since losing part of their vision. This exhaustion is the result of emotional and physical demands that adversely affect our bodies and can impact such things as digestion, sleep, and visual acuity.

I talked with another person about the physical effects of intense stress on those with vision problems. Marcia Applegate is a social worker for the Community Services for the Blind and Partially Sighted, a nonprofit organization in Seattle. She told me that stress is a serious problem among older people who live alone, because they are particularly subject to depression, which is both chronic and debilitating. At its worst, depression can be paralyzing, literally making a person want to roll up into a ball and lie in bed for days. In depression there is often a struggle with self-image and self-confidence. And if someone feels stigmatized by vision loss, this can lead to loss of self-respect and, in turn, depression.

In its own indirect way, depression affects the body by debilitating it. Those who are depressed lack the energy to do anything. Often they want to cut themselves off from the world and not talk with anybody. This can only worsen the problem. We all need interaction—we need the support of other people, and we need physical contact.

The Effects of Stress on Vision

The irony of all this is that the more stressed we are, the more blurred our vision becomes!

When you are under stress, muscles in your body tighten, blood flow to your brain is restricted, and your immune system is weakened. When I asked Dr. Hinton about the effect of stress on eye disease, he gave a slow, careful answer. "If one has a propensity to a particular disease," he said, "stress could certainly bring it out." This, I assume, means that if your genetic inheritance makes you vulnerable to the development of an eye disease, stress could weaken your immune system, making the disease's appearance more likely. This is an important point: excess stress could push you over the edge.

Dr. Hinton offered another, even more interesting observation. He said that during the Cambodian war, many Cambodians developed hysterical blindness. The terrible stress of war effectively made these people blind, even though there was no physical change to their eyes!

This phenomenon of visual impairment due to stress was studied long ago by William Bates, a turn-of-the-century New York ophthalmologist. He found that frustration could cause temporary near-sightedness. He first noticed this with dogs—he showed them meat, then hid the meat behind a curtain. He immediately measured the dogs' vision and found their sight had diminished. In fact, in every case of refractive error in animals and humans, he found a psychological strain in the body, the face, and especially the eyes.

During the preparation of this book, I often noticed increased blurring of my vision when I was tired or upset. My eyes itched, and sometimes I experienced stabs of pain. When I am worn out from a full day's work, I get confused—and when I look out the window, I can't see as well as I could earlier in the day.

For me the blurring is most upsetting of all, because it is like having a veil over my eyes. Women in some cultures wear veils over their faces for modesty's sake—the whole purpose of a veil is to be in hiding, to be shut off from the world. Blurring makes me feel shut off from the world in the same way. And being cut off from the world is a lonely feeling!

Dr. Hinton also talked about the subconscious workings of the eyes and the body. If people watch a movie with images on the border of the screen and are asked to describe what they saw on the edges, they won't remember anything, but the contents may reappear in their dreams. They actually saw the border of the movie—it got recorded—just not consciously. This same thing happens when you experience a stressful situation. You record it subconsciously, and later, when enough stress has built up, it affects your physical health by tiring your eyes or your immune system.

Stress can corrupt your thinking, too. If you are angry or anxious or depressed, you will have a hard time focusing your attention. If you have had a lot of stress in your life lately, this could also affect your ability to pay attention to what you are looking at. In this indirect way, your visual acuity will become worse.

If stress is one of the worst enemies of vision and you do not find relief from stress, then being emotionally upset can actually cause your vision to deteriorate. If, day after day, little frustrations beset you with despair, your visual acuity will begin to reflect that despair.

Ways to Relieve Stress

The three small demons worry, fear, and stress can do you more harm than a fall or accidentally burning or cutting yourself. Burns and bruises heal in a matter of days; stress wounds do not heal unless you take conscious steps to reverse the process.

Coping styles vary from person to person. Loss always brings into question one's character and the nature of life and the universe, which are different for everyone. The following are suggestions for relieving stress. If one method doesn't work for you, try another!

Prevention

Prevention is the best and least expensive medicine! First, eat three good meals and take a walk every day if weather permits. If the weather is not good, find another form of physical exercise. Avoid stress by using other concrete tips mentioned in Chapters 6 and 8. For example, have a selection of magnifiers handy, at least one in each room. Have pads of paper around to jot down things to remember. Keep a diary or journal and pour into it your sadness, anger, or delight at life or unusual things that have happened; whatever comes into your mind. Pick up the phone and call a friend or loved one. If no one is home, leave a message saying you've missed them.

You may find that you need to change your lifestyle from the hectic, fast-paced life most Americans live to a more relaxed pace, tackling only as many errands and social events as are practical. Take it easy. When you have imperfect vision, it takes a lot more energy to do things. Take naps, talk with friends, and entertain yourself periodically. You can still have a wide range of activities in your life, but pare down the more stressful ones. Depending on the degree of your vision loss, your life might be very different now, so pay close attention to how your body is telling you to change.

I find it important to take time out every few hours to meditate or to take a catnap, regardless of how I feel. This is a way to recharge before I become too exhausted. A daily siesta, as I learned during my years in the Mediterranean, is a very healthful habit.

Explore your thoughts and dreams

Jungian analyst Dr. Hinton suggests that to compensate for the loss of outer vision, a person's inner vision probably increases. One might become very introspective when other activities are limited.

When you are unable to sit down with a book to read, let your thoughts wander, recalling books you have read in the past and ideas that have been discussed on a television or radio program. As these ideas float into your mind, meet them with new ideas of your own. Think about events in your past. Ponder strange dreams you have had.

You might find that deliberate thought is also a good way to relieve the stress in your life.

To work on the restlessness and fears inside you, sit yourself down in a comfortable straight chair and think carefully about the things that worry you. Is there indeed reason for you to be upset about these things? Are they worth fretting yourself sick over?

When you find yourself getting pulled down by stress, talk to your inner self (or selves) in a reasonable and soothing way. Pause for a moment, see things in perspective, and say to yourself phrases like "This, too, shall pass. This isn't going to bring the end of the world, and I'm not going to let it ruin my life." Feel your muscles relax, even your eye muscles.

You might also take note of what your subconscious mind is saying through your dreams. Sometimes they just seem silly, but dreams show that your mind continues working while your body is asleep, and they reflect your hopes and your fears.

Research has shown that everybody dreams. People who say they don't dream are just not remembering their dreams. I keep a pad and pen by my bed to jot down notes about my dreams as soon as I awaken. Often what you think is the meaning of a dream may be something else altogether, but just pondering why you have dreamt can help you to study yourself.

One night I awakened from a vivid dream of driving up a hazardous, winding road on a mountainside with other cars constantly passing mine. In the distance I could see another mountain, cone-shaped with a road winding around it to the top. I thought, "How am I ever going to reach the top of my mountain—it's muddy and raining and there are so many cars!" But then a comforting voice began speaking to me: "Just stay where you are," it said. "Calm down; another driver is coming to help you." So I pulled to the side of the road and looked over at the other mountain in the distance, which was now bathed in sunlight. I woke up hearing that reassuring voice again and seeing the sunny mountain, and that dream has remained vivid in my memory for years.

Only later did I come to understand the dream's meaning in my life. I had been inwardly frightened by a succession of rejections by editors, and that godlike voice was telling me that if I would just have faith, things would turn out all right.

Others can help you handle your fears

Most fears are not as great as we imagine them to be. Despite this, it is important to acknowledge fears you might have. If you have friends with a sensible outlook on life, talk your fears out with them. Ask your friends, "Do you think I'm being silly to cling to such a fear?" If they answer that your fears are legitimate, do something about them! If you are afraid of someone breaking into your home, for example, talk over your fear with your neighbors or a block-watch captain. Pick up the telephone and call them!

Most fears, however, when admitted openly will come to seem much less fearsome than you have made them out to be. If your fear is of total blindness, discuss this openly with your ophthalmologist, with someone at a low-vision clinic, or in a support group. These sensible and supportive people will probably remind you of your many capabilities and all the things you don't need to fear at all.

If you have macular degeneration and fear this will lead to total blindness, rest assured this most likely will not occur because the disease affects only central vision, not peripheral vision. In most eye diseases, there will be a long period when you will still see almost normally, and you will have time to adapt to the changes in your vision. In the vast majority of low-vision diseases only one eye is affected at the beginning, and with one good eye you can do almost everything you did before. This should alleviate your fear so that you may cherish what vision you do have. As the stories from other people in this book demonstrate, no matter what your vision problem, you can have a very satisfying life if you make up your mind to do so.

Meditating

I have always been prone to tension. "High-strung" is the term used to describe me. Over the years, I have tried dozens of relaxation techniques. Sometimes I use a method successfully for awhile, then it slowly wanes and another favorite takes its place. One method that has remained in my life throughout the years is meditation.

In its broadest form, meditation can help you find inner peace; close your mind to the noisy, pushy, competitive characteristics of modern life; and connect you to a spirit deep inside. To learn to meditate, I signed up for a class at a Congregational church. In the course, we were shown how to sit down in a comfortable position and take deep breaths, feeling as calm as possible. We would sit still for 30 minutes or more with our eyes closed, and occasionally our teacher would read soothing quotations in a soft voice.

I had always used meditation in the sense of reflecting in a quiet place such as in church, the woods, or my own home. Now I found myself with 40 other people in a church basement, concentrating on our breathing. I soon found that the method worked. Once I tamed the wild horses of my thoughts and focused on nothing else but my breathing, I could feel relaxation steal through me.

The techniques taught in this course are similar to suggestions on meditation from the Lighthouse in New York for people with low-vision diseases. Their recommendations include these:

• Lift your shoulders to your ears and gently release them. Repeat several times.

- Say to yourself, "Relax your toes. Let all of the tension from your toes drain out of your body and into the ground."

- Hum a mantra—a meaningless syllable or a soothing word—over and over.

These basic techniques can be used anytime. I try to meditate every morning, before bedtime, or during a break in the day. If I need to, I also meditate at night when I am having trouble sleeping. Often I meditate to soothing music, breathing in and out while concentrating on the music.

Meditation has definitely improved my health. At the end of that six-week course of weekly meetings, I was decidedly more serene. It has even improved my sleep. Meditation helps me relax, and when I am relaxed the blurring in my vision seems to wane. I highly recommend taking a course in meditation.

Praying to a spirit

Meditation is really a form of prayer. Both are an attempt to halt and release the tempest of internal, intruding voices and reach down to the innermost one: the God within. Prayer is similar to the telepathy often transmitted by touch or an exchange of glances. Direct it to that mysterious spirit that affects all of us, animals and humans alike. Whatever your religious convictions—or even if you have none—prayer can help.

The exercise in meditation mentioned above could just as well be done as a prayer. First, locate a silent place. There is so little opportunity for complete silence in our modern lives, that first finding a little silence is often difficult. It may help to enter an empty church or to walk within sight of a body of water or a forest, where the eternal forces of nature have a soothing effect and the elements absorb other sounds.

Sit down quietly. Breathe deeply, sucking air into your belly and exhaling slowly. Repeat this eight or ten times. Then reach deep into your heart and pray. My prayer is simple: "Dear God, help me." Use whatever prayer or poem is meaningful to you. The important thing is to reach that inner flame, that mysterious contact with spirit, the force that is God within us all. Once again, feel your muscles relax. An epiphany such as this should relax you into a very calm state.

Relaxing at night

My brother John has a favorite method of getting to sleep. He thinks of the last part of the opera Don Giovanni, which he finds boring, and the boredom does the trick! When I am frazzled and cannot get to sleep, I go into my darkened living room, which for me has the overwhelming sanctity of a church. The darkness in this room is my friend. At times I am even aware of the presence of other entities. I sit down and try my meditation mantra, not blocking out the worries as much as smoothing them.

If this does not succeed in bringing on drowsiness, I may try warm milk with a tea bag of chamomile and mint steeped in it. The microwave warms the milk and a bit of steaming-hot water may be added as well. When this warm fluid flows down my throat, it has a tranquilizing effect and usually I can then fall to sleep. Perhaps this effect is the body's remembrance of mother's milk.

Herbal essences in pills or aromas might help you relax, too. Some people say that the essence from specific flowers tames strident nerves and creates peaceful thoughts that soothe the mind. Ask about these at a health and nutrition center.

Music and painting

William Congreve said that music has charms to soothe the savage breast. Again and again when I am feeling upset, angry, or frustrated,

I have been able to regain composure by listening to music that soothes my soul. My favorite is classical, particularly dramatic or romantic pieces with a preponderance of strings. I played the violin from age five until my early twenties, having begged for a violin even before I could read. Though I don't play anymore, I have a large selection of CDs—violin concerti, symphonies with string melodies, and chamber music—that I listen to when I need to relax. The music helps me to escape from my worries and fears, the wild horses of troublesome thought.

Music is more than sound—it is a rebirth of memories, stirring up ideas and dreams within our individual minds, lessening our tensions, and loosening our tightened nerves. Whatever your particular music love, there must be some kind that you respond to with pleasure.

Today there is wide recognition that the mind and body are interconnected. We can help and perhaps even heal ourselves—if we wish to—by determination and believing. Music aids this process by sending joyous messages throughout our limbs. When I listen to particularly exciting music, I feel a throbbing sweep through my body. If it is glorious violin music, my fingers will even move on imaginary strings.

Our bodies *feel* the power of music if our ears do not hear it. Music vibrations are "heard" even by those who are deaf, and sound waves can be "heard" subconsciously by patients undergoing surgery. Babies born prematurely have even been found to respond to Mozart.

Music can soothe one's daily stresses and even release the anxiety of being ill. I once heard of a man who had a blood clot very near his optic nerve and was treated with his favorite music; his emotional response to this music may have helped loosen the clot.

Music is used regularly in prisons, hospitals, and psychiatric wards for its soothing effect. It puts people at ease and brings them closer together. My good friends Alistair and Julia Black tell of meeting one another on the dance floor many years ago; mutual response to the music brought instant communication of mind and soul. Singing brings people closer in the same way—we see this happen in churches and when crowds join together in singing patriotic or nostalgic songs.

But if you want to sing or dance to release some anxiety, you don't have to do it in a crowd. Sing or dance by yourself and you will get just as much benefit as your body relaxes and you move in response to the rhythm. If you think you don't know how to sing, just hum a tune or whistle. You can also use your voice to help cool down. If you want to scream, by all means, do it. Scream out loud! The point is to use your voice in an energetic way to release tension, no matter what it sounds like.

Painting and drawing can relieve stress, too. Winston Churchill took up painting just for relaxation and his work wasn't bad! At that time, the idea that a statesman could paint landscapes surprised everyone.

I, too, have painted for many years for my own enjoyment. When I had a studio or a large room where I could have both an easel and a typewriter, one would help me with the other. If I were very tired at the end of the day after pounding away at the typewriter, getting to the point where my inspiration had fled, I would begin to paint, just picking up brushes and colors, letting something happen to the canvas. Often when I was very tired, I would start to paint and my tiredness would go away. Painting was a tremendous relief from tension and it put my mind on the beauty of nature around me.

Other relaxation techniques

Here are several other ways to reduce stress:

- Go swimming in a lake or pool. Swimming is a great full-body exercise that is good for the heart and cleanses the body.

- Soak in your own hot-water bathtub or a whirlpool. Hot water is tremendously relaxing.

- When your eyes are strained after a day's squinting through magnifiers, lie down for a few minutes with a cold compress or washcloth over your eyes. This is especially helpful if your eyes burn or itch. The palming eye exercise described in Chapter 8 can also help your eyes relax.

- Get regular professional massages. Many licensed massage practitioners will even make house calls, setting up their portable massage tables in your living room.

- Don't underestimate the power of touch. We Americans are often afraid that touch will be misinterpreted. Touching hands, a hug, and even a kiss can be a way of showing friendliness and can in itself lift people from loneliness to feeling wanted. Some scientists say that touch can heal wounds by inspiring relaxation and improving the immune system.

- Play with animals if you have them. People's blood pressure and heart rate lower as they engage in the simple pleasures of stroking the sleek body of a purring cat or petting a happy dog. If you get a cat, try to obtain it as a kitten—a cat who knows you from birth will respond much better to you, even become your personal companion.

People who lose their sight often expand in other ways. Their other senses take over and help compensate. Watch for this in your own life. Tune in to what you previously tuned out. There is a whole new world of feelings, sounds, and smells outside of the world of sight that are a pure delight. On your daily walks notice how each tree rustles in its own personal way. Open your mind to the smell of fresh-cut grass or cumin spice cooking on your stove. Touch everything—run your fingers over the variety of fabrics in the clothes you wear, and touch the people you know more often, shaking their hands and giving them extra hugs. Be open to the world, and stress-free days will come your way.

CAMEOS

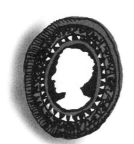

I have felt an unusual connection with some of the people I have interviewed, including **Dr. Clare Buckland,** 83, of Vancouver, B.C. By coincidence, we had cataract surgery on the same day and both discovered the next day that we could no longer read.

As we talked, I found that she and I were both interested in dreams and psychology. Clare began her professional life as an educator, then trained as an analyst when she discovered Jungian psychology. She and Dr. Ladson Hinton started the Analyst Foundation in Seattle. I too have read much about Jungian psychology since the 1940s, and it has been a beacon in my life ever since.

Since being diagnosed with macular degeneration in the spring of 1996, Clare has been unable to read or continue studying. She quit driving that summer and soon moved into a retirement community. In addition to being an analyst, Clare is a writer (another parallel in our lives). She recently published her first book, *Always Becoming: An Autobiography,* and is presently at work on another, *Conscious Living, Conscious Dying*. She uses a CCTV every day and likes books on tape, although most taped book collections do not contain the more professional works she is interested in. Clare found a friend at church who now reads to her. When one of Clare's selections is not available on tape, her friend records the book for her, and they later donate the tapes to the church. Clare values being of service to others in this way.

Clare has always been independent. "The most difficult part of vision loss for me has been to learn to ask for help, she told me. "Now, whenever someone volunteers, I say 'That would be wonderful. Thank you.' When I go out of my way to thank people for their help, it makes a big difference in how I feel, and in how they treat me."

Clare cares for her body as much as her soul. She practices yoga daily, doing floor exercises every morning to "unstiffen" her joints. And every morning she takes a warm shower, ending it with cold water—her own kind of sauna.

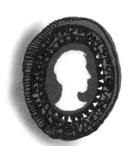 **Tom Morrissey** has struggled with failing vision for at least half his life. He is 40 years old and living in an isolated town north of Denver, Colorado. When I talked with him, I could tell from his voice that he was worried about his future.

It came out that Tom's eye conditions, uveitis and iritis, have no known cause—and his vision changes on an hourly basis. In addition to traditional Western treatments, including laser surgery, Tom has tried acupuncture, herbs, eyewashes, and vitamin supplements, but nothing has improved his condition in any lasting way. Doctors say he is healthy and cannot understand why at his age he has developed these vision problems.

Tom's hobbies are gardening, cooking, and researching sustainable living, but low vision interferes with his enjoyment of them. His wife assists him in his daily life, but she is dealing with her own health problems, so Tom feels very much alone. As I spoke with him about talking books, and what he could find at low-vision clinics and support groups, his voice brightened a little and he seemed to realize there were places where others with vision problems would identify with him. At the end of our conversation he turned quite philosophical. "There must be some lesson in all this, and I'm slowly coming to it."

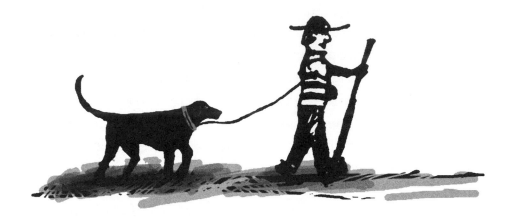

CHAPTER 8

Diet and Exercise

When I was in high school, nutrition was called "domestic science." That was 70 years ago and much has changed since, not only in the appearance, flavor, and food value of what we buy, but also in the rules of nutrition. I have been amused to watch the pendulum of nutritional science swing back and forth.

Your Diet

In my youth, the "perfect foods" were eggs and milk, but now the much-admired Andrew Weil is advising people to avoid these foods. At one time, the very word "protein" was almost magic. People were led to believe that if they ate steaks and hamburgers, they would be strong, healthy, and full of vigor. Now meat products and the saturated fats they contain are viewed by many with alarm.

Even after many decades of changing perceptions, certain principles continue to be respected. The fruits of the earth have been praised from earliest times. In India, as far back as the sixth century B.C., the followers of Buddha abstained from all flesh foods. In the same period in the West, Pythagoras, the Greek philosopher and scientist, opened a school for both men and women where the virtues of vegetarianism were practiced. The diet taught by these wise men of history now has the backing of modern science. Recently, scientists have announced that garden-variety vegetables and fruits also possess chemicals that are healthful for our eyes.

Despite my attention to good nutrition all my life (my diet conforms to the basic philosophy of Epicurus, another of the great Greeks, whose rule was to enjoy everything but in moderation), I still had a small stroke in 1993 and needed carotid artery surgery. This stroke permanently damaged my left eye.

After I found out I had AMD in my right eye, I went to Bill Mitchell, a naturopath and one of the three founders of Seattle's famous John Bastyr University. I wanted to prevent another stroke and to ask his advice on what kind of diet and food supplements would be good for my eyes. Dr. Mitchell is a naturopathic doctor (N.D.), and an easygoing, likable person whom everybody refers to simply as "Bill." I was pleased to find that his approach to diet and vitamins is direct and honest: he believes what you eat can in fact influence your vision.

He also offered a quick way to recognize the produce that is best for the eyes: look for color. In general, look for the fresh fruits and vegetables that are red, yellow, and deep green—the brighter the color, the better. This simple principle is helpful when visiting the supermarket or farm roadside stands.

The Big Four

Dr. Mitchell especially recommends concentrating on "the big four"—carrots, greens, berries, and water. Carrots are good for the eyes because they contain vitamin A. Vitamin A has been found to reduce the likelihood of itching, infection, and cataracts, and it improves night vision. Carrots can be added to almost any meal.

The best greens for the eyes are kale, collard greens, spinach, Swiss chard, turnip greens, romaine lettuce, and bok choy. These contain lutein and a carotein called xanthophyll, which are supposed to protect the tissues of the eye from harmful light and chemicals. The greener the leafy vegetable, the better.

Dr. Mitchell recommends eating all kinds of berries, but at the top of the list are blueberries because they contain the same essential ingredient as bilberries (anthocyanoside). British pilots in World War II ate bilberry jam, swearing that it enhanced their eyesight for night flying and prevented visual fatigue.

A great way to eat blueberries is with yogurt. Blueberries are only in season during the summer, but you can buy them frozen anytime and they're still tasty. Stir them into lowfat or nonfat plain yogurt with crumbled cookies. The cookies will thicken the yogurt, and you can add minced candied ginger and freeze the yogurt if you want a tasty dessert.

According to the 1992 book *Prescription for Cooking and Dietary Wellness,* quality water is important for the eyes because water carries oxygen and other nutrients to cells through the blood and transports waste and poisons out of the body. Simply consuming quality water might help to prevent glaucoma, cataracts, macular degeneration, and many other diseases.

In one study by the Environmental Protection Agency, 200 toxic chemicals were found in water supplies nationwide! If these chemicals enter the bloodstream, traces may stick to artery walls and attract cholesterol, causing the arteries to narrow and restrict blood flow. The smallest arteries are in the extremities of the body, such as the remote parts of the eye, so these locations are especially at risk of complete blockage. At one time, city tap water was often tainted with lead, which, along with other chemicals, can harm the immune system. Consider filtering your tap water—your immune system needs all the help it can get in fighting off threats to your vision.

In addition to drinking *clean* water, older people should probably drink *more* water. As adults, we have a lower percent of reserve body water than do children and often also lose our *desire* for water—our thirst. So we should make it a habit to drink water even when we are not thirsty.

If you want to add something to your water, try bilberry juice—available in bottles at nutrition stores. You can also get your fluids in the form of herbal teas (Dr. Mitchell suggested hibiscus flower tea), but try to avoid caffeine, which can contribute to stress and nervousness, and which, I have found, has affected my vision.

Some Quick Recipes

Here are some recipe hints for vegetable dishes rich in vitamin A. As with all the food suggestions in this book, taste first before adding salt. If you do add salt, start light and add a little at a time.

- *Carrots baked with herbs:* Sprinkle sliced carrots with minced parsley, basil, or mint. Add a pinch of salt and a tablespoon of water. Bake covered in a microwave at high for three minutes or until fork tender.

- *Carrot-potato soup:* Place equal parts carrots and diced white potatoes into chicken or vegetable broth. Add a little diced onion. Simmer until vegetables are tender, then puree in a blender. While hot, add low-fat grated cheese or yogurt, and season to taste.

- *Yam and apple casserole:* Arrange sliced peeled yams and sliced green apples in layers with dried cranberries or raisins and a little brown sugar or maple syrup. Dust with cinnamon. Bake in oven at 350 degrees for about 40 minutes, serving as a side dish with baked ham or roast chicken, or as an entrée in a vegetarian dinner.

- *Roasted carrots:* Thinly slice carrots and spread in a thin layer in a shallow baking tray or dish. Drizzle with olive oil, about 1 Tbs. per pound of carrots. Roast in oven at 400 degrees for about 45 minutes. You can also add strips of red, green, or yellow pepper and coarsely chopped onion. When vegetables are tender, remove from oven and sprinkle with about 1 Tbs. balsamic vinegar. Serve hot or at room temperature.

- *Grated carrots:* Add grated carrots to salads or baked goods such as breads and cookies.

- *Spinach omelet:* This is a quick, easy entrée for one person. Wash chopped spinach, drain well, add to a little olive oil in a small skillet or omelet pan, and sprinkle with salt and pepper to taste. Cook the spinach briefly, then add two well-beaten eggs and cook until the eggs are firm. Turn over with a spatula and slide onto a plate. This is a quick, easy entrée for one person.

- *Creamed spinach:* Wash spinach leaves thoroughly, cook them about two minutes, drain well, and add a creamy pasta sauce that is available in jars. Be sure you check the label for fat content of the sauce and choose one with a low saturated fat content.

- *Swiss chard made with raisins in the Spanish Catalonian style:* Cut the red stems from the Swiss chard, which give it a beety flavor, and cook them in a little water until tender. While the stems are cooking, chop the green leaves and add them to the same pan with 1/2 cup raisins and some salt. Cook until the greens are very tender, about five minutes. Drain thoroughly, add a little olive oil and a dash of vinegar, and serve as a hot salad.

- *Oranges in a tossed salad:* Wash and dry romaine or spinach greens, then crisp in the refrigerator for 15 minutes. Tear up the leaves into small pieces with your fingers. Cut and add orange segments and black olives. Make a dressing of three parts olive oil and one part balsamic vinegar. Sprinkle with freshly ground pepper and add crumbled feta or bleu cheese. Toss well and serve.

Watching fat and cholesterol

Part of eating healthfully is avoiding too much saturated and hydrogenated fats. The body turns these into cholesterol that clogs arteries, slowing the flow of blood to the brain and the eyes and interfering with the nourishing and cleaning of these parts.

Saturated fats include all animal fats and coconut oil and palm kernel oil. Meat, butter, and other dairy products (with the exception of nonfat versions) all contain saturated fat. Coconut and palm kernel oils are commonly used in snack foods such as cookies and crackers.

Hydrogenated fats might sound exotic, but look no farther than margarine and solid shortening. ("Hydrogenated" means that extra hydrogen molecules have been added to liquid fats to make them solid at room temperature. Even "good" oils such as corn and safflower that have been hydrogenated should be avoided.) Be sure to check processed foods at the grocery store for saturated fat and hydrogenated oil content, which by law must be listed on packages.

If you are already on a low-cholesterol diet, stick to it. It can help your eyes. If not, try broiling your foods instead of frying them. In place of butter, use olive or canola oil. These are monosaturated fats, which some experts feel are more beneficial (or less harmful) than saturated fats or polyunsaturated fats (corn oil).

Tofu and seitan are great low-fat protein substitutes for red meats, and are easy to cook with because they absorb other flavors well. You might try these recipe ideas:

- *Tofu in a stirfry:* Start with a minimum amount of canola oil, adding more as you need it. Sauté minced garlic and green onion, stirring until soft and yellow. Add any of the following: chopped bok choy, celery, sliced canned water chestnuts, carrots sliced at an angle, sliced mushrooms or small whole caps, broccoli florets. Stir-fry (in a wok if possible, simply because you don't need to use as much oil) until all ingredients are barely tender. Add chicken or vegetable broth, diced tofu and, if desired, a little diced chicken, lean beef, or fish. Sprinkle with soy sauce and serve with rice.

- *Chunks of tofu in stew:* Add chunks of tofu to a stew or vegetable soup that you have already prepared.

- *Sliced tofu in sandwiches:* Spread peanut butter on bread and top with extra firm tofu. You might also try putting tofu on bread with lettuce and adding salmon mousse, mashed avocado, or egg salad (depending on your cholesterol concerns).

- *Tofu as a dip:* In a blender, combine a garlic clove with olive oil, and add chunks of soft tofu, a squeeze of fresh lemon juice, and spices to taste. Blend until smooth, chill, and spread on wheat crackers.

A good goal is to eat three meals each day composed of a variety of healthful foods. According to Dr. Mitchell, when you miss meals your blood sugar level drops, and this is hard on the body, including the eyes. Good general health will ensure that you can stay active and keep in good spirits.

Fiber

Fiber is another important part of a healthful diet, and there is an enormous variety of fiber-rich foods available. One category is unrefined grains and cereals including wheat, corn, oats, rice, and millet. If you are buying bread, don't be fooled by the words "wheat (or oat, and so on) flour." What you want is assurance that you are getting the unrefined grain so look for "**whole** wheat." Vegetables—including carrots, beets, turnips, broccoli, kale, and cauliflower—are rich in fiber, and most can be eaten raw or lightly cooked. The legume family—including peas, beans, and lentils—is also rich in fiber. Fruits are another good source, especially apricots, apples, and dried fruits such as raisins and prunes. Nuts contain fiber, but limit your choices to unsalted and raw or dry-roasted varieties; they contain enough oil of their own without adding more. Eat nuts in moderation, as they are relatively high in fat.

What does not belong on the list of fiber-rich foods? Grain products made with refined flour, and fruits or vegetables that have been overcooked (which also lessens their vitamin content). Eat foods as close to their natural state as possible—the less processing they go through before they reach you, the better.

Vitamin and Herbal Supplements: Some Pros and Cons

Vitamin supplements are a way to obtain nutrients that our food-intake might not supply. However, I have a few warnings about vitamins before we get into the recommendations.

Food supplements are a huge business—Americans spend some $4 billion on them every year, but not necessarily because of their benefits. Advertisements in mail-order catalogs yell out to us: "Giant Vitamin Sale! Buy 2, Get 3 Free! Free Flashlight with Every Order!" The very fact that it takes these kinds of promises to sell vitamins makes the industry suspect.

The Food and Drug Administration has recorded more than 2,500 adverse reactions and 789 deaths due to supplements. Many of these reactions were attributable to herbal products containing stimulants as additives. The FDA says the side effects from such additives could include heart palpitations, heart attacks, and strokes. This is a great reason to select additive-free vitamins.

Supplements can also cause serious health problems by interacting negatively with some medicines. And even pure supplements can be toxic if taken in excess, because each element in our bodies functions efficiently only when it is in balance with the others.

As surprising as it may sound, the U.S. government barely regulates supplements. Claims of purity, safety, and effectiveness of a supplement need to be filed by companies within 30 days after marketing a product, but these claims are rarely checked by the FDA. Thus there is no guarantee of purity, quantity of active ingredients, or, of course, any beneficial effect. Some attempts are being made to widen the FDA's authority to *demand* proof of health claims and *enforce* quality, but until then we are on our own.

The United States Recommended Dietary Allowance (USRDA) is the closest guide consumers have to understanding what are acceptable doses of supplements. The RDA standard began in 1945 to stop diseases that occur in the absence of certain vitamins. Scurvy, for example, will emerge in otherwise healthy people if their diets severely lack vitamin C, so the RDA for vitamin C was originally set by determining what minimum amount of vitamin C would prevent scurvy.

RDAs have evolved and are updated from current research every five to ten years, but when deciding upon the standard of the RDA for each vitamin and mineral, the U.S. government does not consider what some alternative practitioners believe might help prevent or even cure a disease. The RDA for vitamin A, for example, is based on how much it takes to maintain normal blood cells, not on how much it takes to cure a vision problem. So, if you are considering taking a supplement to try to control or reverse macular degeneration, the government's RDA might be inadequate. The RDA might also be inadequate if one needs to restore depleted vitamin and mineral levels after a lifetime of poor dietary habits, or during the chronic use of medications. In general, intakes of no more than three times the RDA are probably safe, but therapeutic doses of vitamins (10 times the RDA or more) might have detrimental effects on one's health (and one's pocketbook!). If you are considering taking more than the RDA of any vitamin or mineral, you should always do so in consultation with your healthcare practitioner.

Antioxidants

Many research studies have presented evidence that *antioxidant* substances can help prevent heart disease and cancer, as well as cataracts and macular degeneration. To understand the role of antioxidants in the body, we must first talk about free radicals.

Our bodies convert food into energy by using oxygen in a process called *oxidation*. Like any fuel-burning process, oxidation produces toxic byproducts, in this case called *free radicals*. Our bodies also absorb free radicals from outside sources such as tobacco smoke, smog, and pesticides. These substances roam about the body, not only destroying healthy tissue and blocking arteries, but also turning fats and proteins into additional free radicals. Many diseases are associated with free-radical damage, everything from asthma to eczema and, not surprisingly, macular degeneration.

Antioxidants are substances that plants form to protect themselves from free radicals. By eating these plants—also known as fruits and vegetables—we transfer antioxidants into our own bodies and help neutralize the effects of free radicals. In *Stop Aging Now* Jean Carper describes antioxidants this way: "If the free radicals are the thugs of the body, the antioxidants are the police force."

Since macular degeneration is believed to be brought on by free-radical damage in the small arteries of the retina, the Department of Veterans Affairs decided to study the effect of antioxidants on the disease. Their research suggested that taking an antioxidant supplement containing vitamin C, vitamin E, vitamin A, and selenium could slow macular degeneration. Many other studies have come to this same conclusion, but often the studies are weak; either they are small-scale or have not been replicated at other times on human subjects. To date, there is little evidence that taking antioxidants actually results *directly* in the tying up of free radicals that would otherwise do damage, though research is ongoing. For the moment, the evidence seems to suggest that antioxidants can help people with eye diseases.

Dr. Steve Masley, author of *The 28-Day Antioxidant Diet Program* (Custom Printing Company, 1996), and others emphasize getting antioxidants from our diet. In other words, we should be eating more fruits, vegetables, whole grains, and beans—all things we should be eating anyway as a recipe for general good health!

Vitamin A was the first vitamin to be discovered. As early as 1912, studies repeatedly found that the eyes of animals became inflamed and infected when their diets lacked it. A later study that lasted 14 years and involved 50,000 women found a 40% lower rate of cataract surgery among women whose diets were rich in vitamin A, compared with those whose diets lacked the vitamin.

Vitamin A gives us a source of visual purple, a chemical that many studies have found aids nighttime vision. Vitamin A occurs naturally in many foods, including carrots and cod liver oil, and the sun is also important to our bodies' production of the vitamin. The RDA for vitamin A for adults is 5,000 IU; if you take too much, you might get dry eyes, dry skin, and headaches.

In his 1994 book *Natural Prescriptions* (Carol Southern Books), Dr. Robert Giller reports that people who took vitamin C (the RDA for adults is 60 mg) were less likely to have cataracts. While this is another antioxidant that is said to be good for the low-vision diseases, massive doses can harm a person's immune system and promote kidney stones. Besides, as vitamin C is water-soluble, any extra will simply be urinated out of the body and not benefit one's health.

The antioxidant vitamin E has also been found to reduce the risk of cataracts and AMD. Dr. Giller found that people who took about 40 IU (RDA is 8–10 IU) of vitamin E cut their risk of getting cataracts in half, and people who took both vitamins C and E were almost entirely free of cataracts.

Vitamin B is another antioxidant that has been suggested to be an essential nutrient for the maintenance of normal eyesight, but studies are inconclusive. In toxic levels, the vitamin can cause irreversible nerve damage.

Zinc, another antioxidant, is one of the most common trace minerals in the body. It is highly concentrated in the eye, particularly in the retina and tissues around the macula. Zinc is necessary for the action of over 100 enzymes; however, research studies of zinc have been somewhat contradictory. One large-scale study found no reduction of AMD in individuals who reported taking zinc. On the other hand, studies have shown that some older people have low levels of zinc in their blood, either because of poor diet or poor absorption of zinc from food.

The best natural source of zinc is seaweed, but if you decide to take a supplement, pay close attention to how much zinc you already consume and to the way your body reacts to the mineral. Long-term megadoses of zinc can produce a copper or other mineral deficiency because the minerals compete in the small intestine for absorption. Mineral deficiencies can lead to the malfunction of the liver or kidneys. What's more, zinc can suppress the immune response altogether. Dr. McMillan says men who have worked in zinc mines have come down with a variety of illnesses. If the research on zinc has produced any firm conclusions, it is that too much zinc is bad for your overall health.

Again, I recommend that if you want to try any herbal or vitamin therapy, you should do so in consultation with your eye care specialist.

Herbs and other nutrients

Several other supplements may be beneficial to people with eye diseases. Following is a summary.

- *Ginkgo* has been used in Germany and France for depression and anxiety since 1965, but research took off in the early 1980s when French scientists showed that the herb interferes with the chemical responsible for blood clotting. Another French study published in 1988 examined the effect of ginkgo extract specifically on macular degeneration. This double-blind clinical study was conducted with 20 patients over 55 years of age. Ten of the patients received ginkgo extract each day while the other ten received a placebo. After six months, the ginkgo group showed "significant improvement" in acuity of distance vision.

Since blood flow to the retina decreases as we age, our eyes may not be getting the nutrients they need to prevent deterioration of the retina. It is believed that ginkgo relaxes blood vessels, stimulating the circulatory system to carry nutrients to the retina, and helping the brain to comprehend images sent by the eye. It has also been said to reduce itching and swelling of the eyes. Ginkgo overdose, however, can cause skin disorders and headaches.

- My naturopath, Bill Mitchell, gave me a thick, dark purple liquid, which, when diluted in water, tastes a little like lemonade. The liquid is *anthocyanoside,* the active ingredient in bilberry, a fruit extract that that has long been used to improve night vision.

- The *Encyclopedia of Nutrition and Good Health* reports that *zeaxanthin* reduces the risk of AMD. This antioxidant devours free radicals and protects the retina by filtering out damaging light. Zeaxanthin occurs naturally in all deep-green leafy vegetables such as kale, collard, spinach, and mustard greens.

- The *omega-3 fatty acids* found in fish oils might be essential to the maintenance of good eyesight. Like zinc, large amounts of these fats are found in the tissues of the eye, so it has been suggested that frequent servings of steamed, baked, or broiled fish should be included in the diet.

- Researchers from two Universities in Florida showed *lutein* could help in color vision. For this reason, people with retinitis pigmentosa might find this nutrient especially helpful. Lutein can increase the amount of pigments in the retina, which are thought to protect the retina from the harmful effects of light exposure. This nutrient is found naturally in most dark-green leafy vegetables.

- Other things that may help the eyes but lack scientific research to back up their effectiveness include *bioflavonoids,* which are supposed to protect the oils in the eye and are found naturally in vegetables. The herbs *eyebright* and *pot marigold* have been used to soothe irritated eyes that are in pain. These are available in the form of pills, tea bags, eye-drops, and an eyewash.

- My nutritionist Dr. Mitchell told me the Chinese say "the eyes are the sense organ of the liver"—perhaps because the liver cleans the blood and the blood cleans the eyes. The mineral *selenium* helps form a necessary enzyme in the liver, and *milk thistle* and *turmeric* have also been said to be good for the liver and eyes.

All of the vitamins, minerals, and herbs that have been mentioned here are of natural origin, so look first to the fruits, vegetables, and grains that supply them. A tremendous variety of foods is available in better grocery stores—take advantage of it! Don't forget about the more uncommon foods such as guava, apricots, watermelon, pumpkin, okra, and seaweed, which contain antioxidants, B vitamins, zinc, and selenium—as well as other nutrients said to be important to the eyes.

If you feel you must ingest supplements, it might be worthwhile for you to see a nutritionist, dietitian, or herbalist who can closely and objectively monitor the changes your body will go through. As with doctors, make sure any nutritionist you choose is competent and a good listener, not someone who is simply selling as many supplements as possible. Try to minimize the number of supplements you take—maybe everything you need is available in an over-the-counter multivitamin like Vizion, Computer Eyes, Ocu-Vite, Bright-Eyes, or Icap, brands that contain conservative dosages that are generally regarded as safe.

Get Regular Exercise

Next to having a healthful diet, getting sufficient exercise is one of the most important steps you can take to improve your well-being.

Walking and other great forms of exercise

Walking is one exercise all doctors recommend. It helps the digestive system and is a cardiovascular activity that increases the circulation. It is convenient—it can be done in your spare time, in a variety of places.

Try to walk at least one mile a day, weather permitting, and no less than three times a week. After you've mastered this distance, gradually increase it to two miles or more. Keeping to a regular schedule is important. If you find excuses not to go out on your walk, it will get harder and harder.

Mark out a route that does not require crossing a street and that has a shelter for rainy days. A nearby park might be ideal. Some people get their daily walk at malls where they can sit and have a cup of tea if they so desire. In Seattle, seniors can walk in the zoo for a small quarterly fee.

As you walk, keep an even pace and swing your arms. If you are concerned about stubbing your toe or falling because of your vision, carry a walking stick to point the way, and keep your eyes on the path—lifting your gaze periodically to see around you as well.

If you have access to a pool, swimming could be another excellent way for you to improve your circulation. A pool is probably the safest place to swim because on a beach there is a greater possibility of bumping into other people or things.

Aerobic exercise and stretching are also good for your body. Join a group at a health center, or stretch in your own home. Try doing these exercises at a certain time every day, making a habit of it. Dancing, jogging, and other sports (see Chapter 11) are all great exercises as well.

Tai chi and yoga

On two trips to China, I watched old men and women out in the streets in the early morning gently waving their arms and legs. At noontime, factory workers would take a break to go into the street to perform some of these motion exercises. Tai chi, as it is called, is a wonderful method of stretching the limbs and exerting the body to develop strength and range of motion. In the U.S., it is taught in health centers, senior centers, and private clubs, especially on the West Coast. Tai chi can be done almost anywhere—at a beach, in your home, out in the yard—and is quite simple.

Some people swear that yoga is the best exercise in the world. This ancient Hindu practice of bodily discipline comprises a variety of balancing, strengthening, stretching, and breathing exercises performed in a variety of positions. People claim that yoga enhances flexibility and stamina, and relaxes and restores the immune system.

If you are elderly, you should probably avoid inverted postures, such as standing on your head. You might try the following yoga techniques instead. Lie on the floor with your arms outstretched and take several deep breaths. Lift your knees almost to your chest, then lower them to the floor to your right side (only as far as they go naturally). After a few seconds or as long as you can hold this comfortably, return your knees to the center and lower them to the left side. This will stretch and develop strength in your upper leg and stomach muscles. While you are on the floor, try making "snow angels"—the ones children do. Spread your arms and legs wide, then bring them back in to touch each other.

Acupressure, Massage, and Reflexology

Acupressure and *acupuncture*—traditional Asian techniques wherein points on the body are stimulated to relieve pain or regulate a body function—are great for the circulation. In acupuncture, needles are used to stimulate the body; in acupressure, fingers are used. Acupuncture is costly and insurance probably won't cover it; acupressure you can do yourself.

My friend **Fern Kennedy** is the person who first guided me to acupressure. Fern was a successful photographer and teacher until she developed AMD and her sight became so bad she could not focus her camera. She found an acupuncturist who treated her with acupuncture and also showed her how to treat herself with acupressure massage for 15 minutes every morning. After a few weeks, Fern suddenly noticed she could read the time on her watch and the advertisements on television. Her doctor measured her vision with the wall chart and it had, in fact, improved. Fern said acupressure and acupuncture also improved her ability to recognize her friends.

I went to the same clinic Fern did and have found acupressure exercises to be very helpful when my eyes are tired and strained. Apparently, similar eye exercises are used by schoolchildren in China on a daily basis. I have described below the method of acupressure that Fern and I use to improve our vision and relieve tension.

Use acupressure twice a day, once in the morning and once in the afternoon. Make sure your fingernails are trimmed and your hands are clean before you touch your face, and keep your eyes closed. (Never rub your eyeballs—this can spread germs and it has been found to be a risk factor for astigmatism.) Sit with your elbows resting on a table. Rub lightly and slowly until each area becomes a little sore, but do not press excessively.

- With your fists closed, press between your eyebrows with your thumbs for a count of ten, then gently massage.

- With your forefingers press on spots just above the pupil on each eyebrow. Hold for a count of ten, then briefly massage.

- At the outer end of each eyebrow, press your forefingers at the tender spot there on the skull, count to ten, and then massage.

- Press your forefinger or your thumb at a spot just below the pupil of each eye on your cheekbone, then massage.

- On the top of your forehead, press your thumbs against the most tender spots on skull. Count ten and massage.

- With thumb and forefinger, pinch five points along each ear, from the top of the outer ear down to the lobe. Repeat several times.

- Resting your fingers above your ears, press your thumbs to
the base of your skull and count to ten, then massage gently.
If this causes too much pain, simply massage the back of
your neck with your fingers.

Massage is a wonderful way to promote the free circulation of
blood and to relax. Dr. Mitchell even suggested getting a massage
once a week, concentrating on the scalp, face, and neck, to improve
circulation to the eyes. One of the secretaries who works in Dr.
Mitchell's office was in a car accident that left her with a very stiff
neck and vision loss to the point of having to wear glasses. However,
after a series of treatments by a special chiropractor who adjusted
and massaged her neck, she no longer needed to wear glasses. Many
massage therapists use oils, but one can do dry massages simply by
lightly brushing fingers over the skin, which is also a good method
of increasing circulation. Call a local massage school in your area for
a referral to an experienced therapist.

Reflexology is a kind of acupressure on the feet that has been
used to treat diseases. The theory behind reflexology is that each
spot on the soles of the feet is linked with another part of the body,
and massaging a particular spot will stimulate the corresponding
body part. The very center of the sole of the foot is said to corre-
spond to the eyes. Here are a few more massages:

- With your hand one palm length above your anklebone on
your shin, press your fingers into a tender spot next to the
leg bone ten times. Repeat with the other leg.

- Press the bottom of your foot directly beneath the arch in the
most tender spot and massage. Massage your entire foot up
and down from back to front, repeating with the other foot.

- Lastly, stand up and gently pound the middle of your back
with your fists several times to "wake it up."

It's curious to think of doing something to your feet or your back to help with your eyes, but if nothing else this will help your whole body to relax.

The Bates method for the eyes

Turn-of-the-century ophthalmologist William Bates believed that if we want to strengthen our eyesight, we should not rely on glasses. He believed they are a crutch we depend on that actually *inhibits* accurate vision. After studying animals and humans for many years, he concluded that poor eyesight is a result of long-term stress and a limited range of vision, so he created a regimen of eye exercises to relax the eyes and stretch their range. Nearly a century later, his method has once again become quite popular.

The Bates method can help you develop your peripheral vision and help your eyes adjust to various intensities of light and negotiate between near and far targets. Each of your eyes should benefit from his method—both the one affected by disease and your better eye. The exercises, which should be performed without contacts or glasses, should help your eyes work together in a balanced way. I find them relaxing not only for my eyes but for my whole body.

• The first exercise is called *palming*. Sit comfortably on a chair at a table. Place your elbows on the table, and cover each of your closed eyes with a cupped hand so as to block out all sources of light. Do not apply any pressure to your eyes—just make sure you see the blackest black possible. Imagine a very dark place, like a cave or a secluded beach at night. Slowly remove your hands, then steadily open your eyes. The theory behind palming is that when we eliminate all outside sources of light, and are relaxed, our eyes are strengthened, thereby enabling us to see finer details and brighter colors in normal conditions. It is recommended that you carry out this exercise for at least five minutes per day.

• *Scanning* involves standing outdoors—or indoors near a window that has a wide, distant view. Start at one end of the horizon—the farthest you can look to the left by turning only your head—and gaze as far out as possible. Gently turn to the right until you are looking at the other end of the horizon. Scan back and forth, stopping from time to time to notice what objects in the distance you can see clearly.

• To perform the *focusing* exercise, fix your gaze on a nearby object, then move your gaze to an object that is far away and hold this focus for a few seconds. Allow your gaze to move again to an object that is closer to you and focus on it for another moment. Now raise your finger in front of your eyes and focus on one particular point on it. Still focusing on your finger, move it near and far. Notice when you can see it clearly and when it begins to fade into a blur. For this exercise, be sure you are relaxed and that you are focusing only on a small area, not necessarily seeing perfectly.

• Dr. Bates does not mention an exercise for peripheral vision, but for people with macular degeneration, this may be one of the most useful exercises of all. Move your eyeballs so you are looking as far to the right as you can. Now look down, then to the left as far as you can. Complete the circle by looking up. Repeat a couple of times. You can also turn your head to the right while looking back toward the left, and vice versa.

Don't skip your eye exercises just because you are tired or in a hurry. It's the day-after-day exercising that counts. I frequently do these exercises in my living room, but they can easily be done in the bathtub, on the bus, or while taking a walk—so do them!

The Bates method allowed my friend Alma Romero to bolster her peripheral vision enough to be able to read, and Dr. McMillan told me that despite my trouble with direct vision, my peripheral vision was strong enough that I could drive a car if I so wished. However, in today's hazardous traffic, I am content to let others do the driving.

CAMEOS

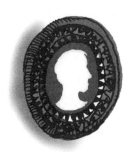

One person who has found bilberry helpful is **Vernon Work,** 83, of Seattle. Vernon had dry AMD in his right eye for ten years, and the day after his birthday two years ago Vernon found he had wet AMD in his left eye. Vernon received laser treatment and in four to six months his vision had stabilized, but he still could not see more than three feet away. A friend from church who also had an eye problem suggested he try taking bilberry to better his vision. After seeking the advice of several ophthalmologists, Vernon thought there was a chance that bilberry would improve his vision.

After taking a capsule a day for about four months, Vernon's vision improved dramatically: instead of only being able to see objects three feet away, he can now see up to 30 feet away. Vernon feels inspired to continue the experiment with the herb. His advice to others is, "Don't program yourself to get old before your time!"

A friend in Evergreen, Colorado, told me about **Evelyn Skinner**. My friend mentioned that Evelyn had had macular degeneration for four years and was still skiing. When I talked with Evelyn later she told me she had formerly lived in McLean, Virginia, only a short distance from Arlington where I used to live. While in McLean, her two favorite sports were swimming and ice skating (a sport she taught over several decades), depending on the season.

Evelyn's boundless energy provoked her friend at the *Washington Post* to write a parody article that he privately printed under the *Post*'s nameplate. The headline read, "Bush names Evelyn Swindler to Replace Watkins as Energy Secretary."

Her energy is equally astonishing to her new neighbors in Evergreen. After the death of her first husband, she took the opportunity to move to Colorado because she had always wanted to ski. She took her first lessons at the age of 65.

She attends church regularly and it was here that she met her second husband. She told me that a certain attractive man always seemed to be sitting in the pew with her. Before long, she found this wasn't accidental. It turned into a romance, then marriage. Now she and her new husband ski together, square dance, and walk three miles every day.

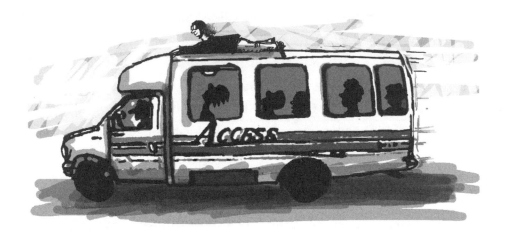

CHAPTER 9

Helpers Are Everywhere

One rainy February afternoon, I set out for a brief walk. I had not been out all day because of the rain, but I needed some fresh air as well as a bit of exercise. I carried my white fold-up cane because of the growing dusk. As I walked along I heard a voice behind me. At first I thought the man was calling someone else, but when I heard his repeated "Ma'am," I turned around. "Are you all right?" he asked. He had noticed my cane and said he thought I might be lost. I assured him I was fine and was nearly home, but I was touched by the helpful concern of this stranger.

This sort of thing happens frequently when I carry my cane. It makes me realize how kind people can be. I have come to think of my white cane as a kind of talisman, an amulet providing help and protection that causes people to react positively and come to my assistance. I believe this attention is not pity, but rather admiration that a disabled person is trying to get along independently.

Customer Assistance

When I go grocery shopping, I usually walk to the nearest shopping center where a good supermarket is located. Fortunately, there is such a market less than a mile from my home and walking there can serve as my daily exercise. Of course I bring my cane with me for crossing streets, and at busy crossings I wait until the green light will stay on long enough for me to cross. Then I hold the cane out so that it is easy for motorists to see. The effect on motorists in both directions is amazing. It makes me feel quite important!

Inside the supermarket I put my fold-up cane into the shopping cart, then ask a clerk for customer assistance. I show my written shopping list to the person assigned to me, who takes me around the market to make my selections. In the produce section I am especially glad to choose my own apples or oranges or whatever produce looks and feels freshest. The assistant usually lets me know when items are on sale, and can suggest easily prepared packaged products. Often, just by being in the market, I am inspired to try something I would not have considered had I phoned in an order or hired someone to shop and deliver groceries to me.

You might be surprised to hear that customer assistance is available for people with low vision in almost every store. Smaller, better shops advertise their customer assistance, but if you need help that is not publicized, don't hesitate to ask. Even in clothing shops, one should be able to get customer assistance for finding and trying on articles.

It might be different at enormous discount stores where one walks between skyscraper-high piles of unopened merchandise with nary a clerk in sight except at the checkout counter. On the off chance that your favorite store cannot help you, ask a friend to accompany you. He or she might be glad of an excuse to do some shopping.

Banks and Telephone Companies

My two greatest headaches are writing checks and making phone calls. Early in my experience with vision loss, I requested help with my checkbook at my bank's local branch. I was shocked to hear, "We don't have the manpower for that." As this branch was part of a large bank with hundreds of employees, this response angered me, especially as they had only recently downsized their employee staff but continued to advertise their superior service! The next day I switched to a bank where I knew I would get help and was pleased to be able to tell the big bank why I had closed my account.

At the small local bank I found altogether different treatment. Here a lovely woman named Carmen Blenman smilingly assured me that she would be happy to help me with my checkbook every month. Still, I try to use as few checks as possible, charging even my grocery bills on a credit card. This way I get a monthly statement showing what each purchase was for, simplifying my bookkeeping.

At tax time there are even more discounts for those of us with limited vision. At least two organizations, Tax Counseling for the Elderly and Volunteer Income Tax Assistance, provide free tax help for the elderly and disabled. Most senior centers and libraries have contact with these organizations, and the Internal Revenue Service knows where this type of assistance is made available. The IRS also offers discounts on federal taxes for those over 65 and for those who are legally blind. People over 65 and legally blind get a double discount! There may also be a discount on state and local taxes; ask your regional representative about this.

As for my other great headache, phone calls, I am grateful to our local phone company, U.S. West. Visually disabled people can get free directory assistance within their region, and the company will even dial a telephone number so you don't have to fumble with buttons. I appreciate this regional service all the more because the great AT&T does not provide it for long distance—in fact, trying to get telephone numbers through their service can be very exasperating. We who have visual difficulties should demand more from the giants!

Transportation Options and Benefits

Taxicabs are really a lifesaver for the trip home after I have shopped for groceries. All seniors and disabled people get the benefit of half-price taxi "scrip" through Seattle's Metro Transit. Because of my low vision I can get $60 worth of cab rides a month for $30. Plus, since I do not live far from the market, the cab fare is reasonable—much less costly than paying for delivery—and the cab drivers are nearly all thoughtful and kind. I like to converse with the drivers and am often very impressed with their knowledge about what's happening in the world. By the time we reach my address, we are acquainted and usually the driver offers to carry my grocery bags to the door—sometimes even up the steps to my apartment.

Seattle offers even more transportation options for people with disabilities. This includes very low priced bus fares for seniors and the disabled, and a van service (called Access) to and from people's homes. The charge is minimal, under a dollar. Sometimes the wait for the van seems interminable and on rare occasions it fails to appear, but for people who want to go to the same place day after day and week after week, the vans are a wonderful service. Most large cities have similar services for people who are elderly or disabled in some way.

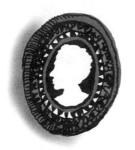

One woman I talked to makes regular use of the van service. **Peggy Marshall**, who is in her sixties, has worked for years for a local drugstore chain but because of macular degeneration she could no longer write invoices. Peggy's employers rewarded her loyal service by giving her a position in which she didn't have to perform this duty, and she began taking the van service to work three days a week. On the other days of the week she uses the same van service to go to the park, to her hairdresser, to meetings, or to visit friends.

Volunteers

Most of the people I have talked with have a son or daughter who helps them with errands and tasks around the house. If you're looking for help, ask among your family first, especially family members who live near you. Don't forget all the little chores they could help with—like opening bottles or fixing a TV or VCR. If your immediate family live too far away, maybe they know another relative or a friend who lives near you and can volunteer.

You might also find a helper right next door or across the street who would be happy to come and read to you now and then or take you shopping. If you live in a city or suburb, you might have a block-watch captain who could tell you of someone who is personable and service-minded.

Sometimes when traveling in the various buses and taxicabs, one finds friendly, sympathetic people who would be happy to help you out in your personal life. When I was badly in need of someone to read to me, I mentioned this problem to a cab driver and he said he would be happy to volunteer for me during his off-hours, since he lived nearby. One of my neighbors became alarmed when I told her I invited him to come and read for me, but I myself have traveled through many countries and have never been bothered by the strangers with whom I struck up conversations. Since I had already invited the cab driver, I welcomed him into my home and found him to be intelligent, interesting, and good at reading—just as I expected. It turned out his hours were too irregular for me, but this proves you can find volunteers anywhere.

Senior centers in every city usually have an extensive network of people and groups such as dance and game clubs, and it is often possible to find volunteers through this network, even if you are not a senior. Professional and social clubs like the Rotary Club and the Kiwanis or an ethnic organization you belong to could provide great opportunities, and churches and other houses of worship are usually very kind to their members. One or more of the above organizations will surely be able to assist you in finding volunteers for reading, driving to doctors' offices and the hairdresser, and even doing the dishes and weeding the garden.

If you just aren't having any luck in finding volunteer help, you might try advertising, preferably in a newsletter of a local organization or in a local community paper. In your ad, simply say that you have low vision and are looking for someone who can come to your aid on a volunteer basis. Here again, family and friends could be helpful. They could screen volunteers to weed out any who might prove more tiresome than helpful or who might not be reliable.

If you open your own heart and mind and try to wipe out your prejudices, you might discover some very interesting people out there. Novelists say that everybody's life story is a potential novel, and if you yourself have had an interesting life, that should be remembered and mentioned as you search for volunteer help. These volunteers would not only be doing you a service, they might find you interesting and be curious about what it's like to be visually impaired.

Support Groups

I met an interesting woman named Carin Mack at a lecture on cataract surgery that was given at one of the four low-vision support groups she leads. Carin is a slender, energetic administrator who glows with enthusiasm for her work, planning interesting lectures for the support groups and urging people to come to the social gatherings simply to exchange experiences, both good and bad.

Support groups for low vision fulfill quite a different function than low-vision clinics. While low-vision clinics sell devices and give eye exams, support groups are free social get-togethers for people with low vision—whether due to cataracts, macular degeneration, or any other eye disease. Support groups perform an educational function, supplying those who come to the meetings with printed material about their particular eye disease and how to cope with it. Occasionally there will be lectures by physicians and others in the medical field. Each group has a unique style and personality reflecting the neighborhood in which it meets, and they vary in size and social and financial resources.

When I attended a group of Carin's that met in a senior center, all 20 of us sat around a large table in a sunny room. Carin knew many of the people already and quickly made the rest feel at home. She went around the circle asking if people had anything interesting to report.

Each of those present told about things he or she had learned, tricks or easy-to-obtain devices that might be useful for all of us.

One man showed off an interesting pair of binoculars that looked like opera glasses. He demonstrated how he could wear them over his regular glasses and hang them around his neck when not in use. When, after the meeting, he permitted me to look through them, I was impressed with how well they magnified objects some distance away; I had been looking for something like them for awhile.

After several people had offered their news and tips, one frail-looking woman spoke up in a trembling voice. This was her first visit to a support group, so at first she found it hard to speak. Her story was horrifying. She had gone to an ophthalmologist for cataract surgery and specified on a questionnaire before her operation that she was allergic to anesthetics. She also told both the nurse and the surgeon verbally about her allergy. Nevertheless, the surgeon used a local anesthetic for her surgery and that night, alone in her apartment, she woke up with a violent fit of vomiting. Her vision did not improve, so she returned to the clinic a few days later and found that she had macular degeneration. As she expressed her pain and fear her voice became louder and more bitter.

It was clear that everyone in the group was shocked at her terrible experience. I, too, live alone, so I could imagine how disturbing it must have been for her—getting sick and not having anyone there to help. We were all very sympathetic, and everyone offered advice. I could see that gatherings of this sort allow people to share personal ordeals and feelings with others who can relate.

At the end of the meeting, we received information about coming events for people with low vision. I was impressed with how well most of the people in the group had adjusted to their vision problems.

To find a low-vision support group in your community, first ask your ophthalmologist. If he or she does not know about one, don't be surprised. Unfortunately, few eye specialists seem to consider this their responsibility. Try calling the Lighthouse in New York City (800-334-5497). They have a listing of low-vision centers in the nation by city and state, and the centers will probably be able to direct you to support groups. In your search for a support group, it is important to find one that suits you, with people of similar interests and temperament. If a certain group does not feel right for you, try another.

Making New Friends

Attending a support group is a great way to make new friends who understand your daily stresses, and these people can lend support even outside the group you attend. I have met several friends when they first served me as volunteers. One woman was referred to me by Community Services for the Blind and another by the neighborhood senior center. Anytime I needed readers, they were on my list of volunteers, and when they visited we found we had many common interests!

When trying to meet new friends, it's OK to talk to strangers, just proceed with caution. Whether standing in line in a store or walking near others in the park, you can start up conversations with anybody who looks interesting. Try to find some common interests and stay bright and cheerful. Find an excuse to mention what your chief passion is or has been all your life; this in itself might open up a new avenue of mutual interest. Elise Matthews, whose story is told in Chapter 5, met her husband at a bus stop, after a friendly exchange. It is wise, however, to gather as much information as you can about strangers before exchanging addresses. If someone comes up to you and asks impertinent questions, be friendly—but stay on your guard.

The Lighthouse National Survey on Vision Loss revealed that a lot of normally sighted people feel "awkward or embarrassed" because they do not know how to behave around people who have vision problems. This feeling is even more common among people who interact with a close family member who is visually impaired. It is not surprising then that people often address the companion of a visually disabled person instead of addressing the disabled person directly—for example, a waiter might ask the companion, "What does she want to order?" You don't want this to happen—you want people to talk with you directly. Here are a few suggestions for putting others at ease:

• **Turn your head toward people**—in turn, they will speak directly to you.

• **Present yourself with confidence.** Be the first one to speak. Say hello. Introduce yourself.

• **Smile**. Remember the song, "A smile is your umbrella on a rainy day"? It's amazing how far a simple smile can take a person in life.

• **Be positive and use humor.** Talk about the vision you have, not what you don't have. One person with macular degeneration said, "I don't see dust and no one wants me to do windows." Laugh when you say to people, "My hearing is OK so you don't need to talk so slowly."

• **Educate, don't criticize.** Let's face it, some people with full sight have no idea what it's like to be visually impaired. Explain to people how your vision is affected. Tell people how you would like to take their arm if you need help walking.

In general, be positive and self-assured and show your interest in other people, and they will be more likely to respond to you. Ask lots of questions about people's lives—people like to talk about themselves! Once you have established a friendship, you can ask your new acquaintances for help when you need it.

CAMEOS

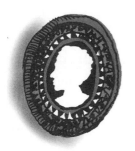

Annabelle Seidman of Falls Church, Virginia, was diagnosed with AMD ten years ago, but she doesn't let anything slow her down. She is active in many organizations, including regular meetings with a support group for people with low vision. To get to her meetings, she has to take a subway and transfer three times, but she has learned how to do this and now traveling long distances doesn't bother her. She is still working as both a supervisor for one of the branches of a government service organization for the blind, and as a consultant for a vocational rehabilitation agency in Arlington, Virginia, called Independence. When she is not working, Annabelle enjoys the radio program "The Listening Ear," which reads the newspaper over a special frequency.

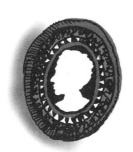

Barbara Montgomery, of Chanhassen, Minnesota, is 77 and legally blind in both eyes from dry macular degeneration. Barbara has lived a life of creativity with her hobbies of writing and watercolor painting, and has always been helping others. She was the director of a women's center for many years and once worked at a crisis hotline for teenagers. Even though her independence is limited by low vision, Barbara loves to volunteer and share information with others. A few years ago she received funds from the "Thanks Be to Grandmother Winifred Foundation" to research and distribute resource information to women with AMD. She continues in this spirit by giving talks to groups at senior centers and senior expositions on the subject of macular degeneration. Barbara misses being able to drive and has lost some of the independence she once had, but her son and grandson visit her regularly to help her with reading and transportation.

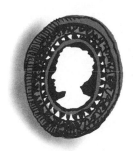 **Soo-Z Stein** of Washington, D.C., is a senior who doesn't let AMD stop her from playing golf twice a week. When her vision began to deteriorate, she switched to orange golf balls and has her husband or caddy point her in the right direction. She also gets exercise by using a treadmill regularly.

Soo-Z found out about her macular degeneration 50 years ago when her doctor didn't even know what it was. Nowadays she serves on the board of the Low Vision Information Center in Bethesda, Maryland. She especially enjoys the time she spends on this project because she feels good about helping other people with vision problems. This nonprofit center provides all kinds of brochures and literature on macular degeneration; it is arranged as an apartment set up with labels and markers so people can see how to use low-vision aids in a home-like setting. The information center is supported entirely by donations and has become very popular in recent years—people from as far away as Europe come to see what it offers.

Soo-Z does her own housework and cooking and has adopted a dog from a local animal shelter for company during the day. "There's always something to keep me busy, and that's the name of the game," she says. "And if I can help somebody else . . . and keep a smile on my face . . . that's good, too."

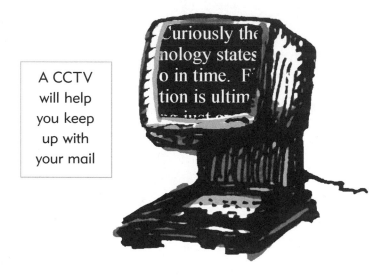

A CCTV will help you keep up with your mail

CHAPTER 10

The Wonders of Technology

As I start this chapter, I am also beginning a new chapter in my life. I am practicing on my new computer that announces aloud what I am writing as I hit the keys. The software is called JAWS, and I call the male voice I hear "Charlie."

Sometimes I get annoyed with Charlie because he announces all the punctuation and spaces I type and has a hard time keeping up with my speedy touch-typing. Because I cannot read from the monitor anymore, or see where the mouse is pointed, I have to practice new keyboard commands to maneuver through the programs. I am learning a new language. Eventually, I will be able to do everything I used to do on the computer, with vocal direction to steer me where I want to go.

Another new wonder on my desk is a scanner and software program with the enchanting name of OpenBook (Arkenstone). When I first saw this demonstrated, I was amazed at the scanner's ability to read printed material by columns, going from the bottom of one column to the top of the next. This program is limited to printed text, however—it will not let me read handwritten letters or postcards—so I must ask friends who send cards to type their messages if they can.

The system actually has many voices besides Charlie's—if you'd rather listen to a Myrtle or a Spike, you can. Like the keyboard commands, however, these synthesized voices take some getting used to. I feel as though I am trying to understand a heavy foreign accent, but eventually even the synthesized voices seem almost human. In time I hope to feel comfortable reading my mail and magazine or newspaper articles with all my new machinery.

A Few Gadgets to Get You Started

This new talking technology of mine will probably never completely replace my closed-circuit television (CCTV), described in Chapter 5. The great advantage of this viewing machine over the scanner and talking software is that I can pencil changes on the printed sheet and read them immediately. The talking software cannot read handwriting, and the time required for it to scan can be painfully long even for brief texts. What's more, the CCTV is simple—you turn on the switch and read the magnified print. The scanner and computer software, on the other hand, are mazes that must be navigated by keyboard.

It is possible to buy CCTV software that turns your personal computer and scanner into a device that enlarges text like a CCTV. Some CCTVs are portable and use a handheld camera that is passed over the text to be enlarged. I have seen these in the various low-vision catalogs. Such units are probably less expensive than buying a whole new CCTV because they are smaller and hook up to a TV or a computer screen you already own.

Some gadgets that enlarge text and images are so portable that they can be worn over regular eyeglasses! One such system is called the V-max—a tiny color camera and display system that uses digital images to capture and enlarge text and objects. I found a description of this device in the Autumn 1997 "Low Vision Viewpoint," a newsletter of Community Services for the Blind and Partially Sighted in Seattle. This device works something like a camcorder. With the V-max glasses, you view a tiny television image about the same size as the image you would see in a camcorder—except on the V-max, you are viewing the pictures, not recording them. The V-max can enlarge any image, from labels up close to road signs in the distance, but there is a catch: it costs $4,000.

The Resources section lists several catalogs that sell many devices that talk in synthesized voices. Most catalogs sell talking scales for about $80 and thermometers for $60 that keep numbers in memory and will announce aloud your weight or temperature. These can be very good for people who cannot see small numbers but have to check their weight or temperature on a regular basis for medical reasons.

These catalogs also sell wristwatches and clocks that tell the time out loud. Instead of trying to read near-microscopic marks on your watch, why not get one that does the work for you? The watches talk either at the push of a button or automatically at the top of the hour. My talking wristwatch has not only proved invaluable, but also is good for a laugh in mixed company. Suddenly they hear a strange voice—"It is now 2:15 P.M.!"—and look for the speaker. Similarly, talking alarm clocks will wake you in the morning by announcing the time. And talking calculators make balancing your checkbook a whole lot easier. These kinds of gadgets are priced $15 and up.

The LS&S catalog sells little devices, worn on your belt or just held in your hand, that vibrate if you are about to bump into something. They work by sending out an invisible light to detect barriers like telephone poles or walls, then warn you with a vibration that you can distinctly feel against your skin.

These amazing new technologies, which weren't available just a few short years ago, are improving with each passing year.

Computer Software and Hardware

Personal computers have seen a lot of innovations in recent years, both in software and hardware that have opened all kinds of doors for those of us who have lost some of our vision. First I should explain what is meant by software and hardware. In very simple terms, "software" refers to programs, or sets of instructions, that tell the "hardware," or physical equipment, what to do.

Software

Some software comes with a computer and forms the basic "brains" or instructions that run the computer. This is called an "operating system." Other software programs, available on computer disks or CD-ROMs, allow a computer user to perform more specialized functions such as word processing and accounting. These are called "applications." (See Resources for addresses of the companies that sell low-vision software.)

Concerning the cost of computer equipment and software: If the prices listed put you off, don't despair. Help is available for those with special needs. The first place to check is your state's Department of Services for the Blind. The Lions Club has money available for people who can demonstrate need. Some funding might also be available through Medicaid or local nonprofits helping people with low vision. One such agency in Seattle is the Community Services for the Blind and Partially Sighted. National groups that refer people to funding sources are the National Rehabilitation Information Center and the Alliance for Technology Access. If, after contacting these organizations, you still have not found sources of funding, just keep asking around; something is bound to turn up somewhere.

Software programs for people with low vision fall into several categories, which are described below.

- *Keyboard enhancers:* These programs change the keyboard to make it easier to use for people with low vision and other disabilities. HandiWORD (Microsystems Software, $350) is one such software program. People with low vision tend to make typing mistakes, and this program corrects many such mistakes and stops accidental repetitions of letters. The program actually anticipates what letter will come next in a word and what word will come next in a predictable phrase. For example, the phrase "if I am late" will probably be followed by a phrase beginning with the word "then." If you make a mistake and type "theb" instead of "then" (because "b" is right next to "n" on the keyboard), the program will correct this automatically. This makes it easier for people with low vision to type accurately.

- *Screen enlarger programs:* These programs make words on a computer screen bigger so people with low vision can see them. Screen enlargers work with most word processing programs, making dialog boxes and text taller and wider. At least nine of these programs are on the market, ranging in price from $20 to $2,500. Slimware Window Bridge is one of the more popular versions (Syntha-Voice Computers, $600).

- *Screen translators:* This software turns normal text into braille or speech. Several versions of this program are available, but the most popular is JAWS for Windows (Henter-Joyce, $800), which translates screen information into spoken words. It comes with a set of cassette training tapes. Having been a touch-typist for years, I find this program relatively easy to use.

- *Voice recognition programs:* This software adapts to your particular voice and vocabulary, "understands" you better and better each time you speak, and then acts on your spoken instructions. These programs range in price from $50 to $1,000. Dragon Dictate for Windows (Dragon Systems, $400), one popular voice recognition program, features a dictation system that lets you control most Windows programs—even the mouse—entirely with your voice. You don't have to touch the keyboard at all if you don't want to, or you can use both voice and keyboard.

- *Optical character recognition (OCR) programs:* These can transfer printed text from magazines or letters onto the computer for a word processing program or can allow a voice synthesizer to read it aloud. If you wanted to, you could scan in a magazine article with a scanner and an OCR program, have JAWS read it out loud to you, edit out the boring parts, and then send the article to your friend. Amazing, isn't it? One of the popular programs that performs OCR is OpenBook (Arkenstone, $900). OpenBook can translate up to 95% of information into speech, but in addition to buying this software you must also purchase a scanner, the hardware needed to read text into the computer. Scanners are available for under $100.

Most software programs for people with low vision are just now going through a refinement process that other software has undergone for the last decade. As time goes on, software for optical enhancement will only become more sophisticated. For instance, not very long ago voice recognition and optical character recognition programs were not very accurate. Today these programs interpret words and letters *in context*. Optical character reading software now knows it is most probable that the third letter of a three-letter word that begins "th" is "e," not "f," so it prints an "e" for you.

Other aspects of computer technology also need to improve to meet the needs of people with low vision. Judy Schnitzer does marketing over the internet for the Macular Degeneration Foundation. Her work brings her in contact with many Web sites, most of which don't work very well yet with software programs designed to read aloud their contents. Judy is consulting with companies to make their Web sites accessible.

Hardware

Hardware is the physical equipment needed to operate software programs. Most of the software described above does not need expensive or special hardware to run. Normal desktop computers will do, but the standard for what is "normal" in hardware changes every six months or so.

There are two important laws in the computer world. One is that whatever you buy will be instantly "obsolete," but only in the sense that something newer is available out there. Whatever you buy will most likely continue to fill your needs and work well. The second law is that as time goes by in the computer market, prices go down and functionality goes up. The bottom line is, get a computer that does what you need it to do and do not worry that next month something more exciting will be on the market. My guess is that all those clever engineers and marketers want to keep merchandise moving, so they are always creating new products.

You should be prepared to spend about $5,000 if you want a complete setup with adaptive programs. When I acquired my system in early 1998, it came with the following components:

- Keyboard, monitor, and speakers

- Windows 95, JAWS, and OpenBook software

- Scanner

- DECtalk unit with headphones (see description below)

- Sound card and driver

Your keyboard should have large letters and raised dots to keep your fingers where they belong. Clear stickers with raised dots or fluorescent stickers can mark the keys you use the most often. The advantage of clear stickers (available at low-vision clinics) is that the letters underneath are still visible.

DECtalk is the brand name of a device that translates computer text into speech; it is about the size of a cellular phone and can sit next to your computer. DECtalk is the best translator on the market today and the one Stephen Hawking, the renowned astrophysicist with ALS (Lou Gehrig's Disease), uses to communicate.

When shopping for computer equipment, go to a store that has several computers on display that you can test out. Various devices can be combined to assist with tasks. No single electronic device suits everyone; what works for others may not work for you.

In purchasing a computer and software, the first thing to do is to determine *your* needs: what exactly do you want to be able to do? Decide on your priorities, then shop around for the best deal. Maybe you can buy some of your equipment used. Check classified ads, or ask people at the low-vision clinic if they know of anyone who no longer needs their computer.

If you don't know much about computers, get advice from someone who does. If possible, have that person with you when you talk to the salespeople. Don't let salespeople sell you expensive machines that will not really make your daily life better, and pay close attention to the service the salespeople claim they will provide. Does the product have a parts and labor guarantee? How much training on the new equipment will be provided? Will the trainer drive to your home, or will you need to travel to them? Remember that the State Services for the Blind may be able to tutor you on many of these programs. They may also help with funding under special circumstances and according to your needs.

Wonderful Things Lie Ahead

New and extraordinary devices are appearing on the market so fast we can scarcely keep up.

A virtual retinal display (VRD) is like the V-max described earlier—it is a color camera and display that uses digital images to capture and enlarge text or objects. But there is one giant difference in the VRD: it uses "virtual reality" technology. In a normal display, like a television or the V-max, a *real* image is projected onto a screen, and a person watches that screen with light bouncing off it. *With the VRD, no real image is ever produced.* The device shines a low-power laser into the eye and forms images directly on the retina. The person never actually sees anything outside the eye.

A person whose macula has deteriorated could not use the VRD as it works today, but it is possible to combine the VRD with other technology to bend the image so it will sidestep the macula and land on healthy retinal tissue. Developers at the University of Washington in Seattle are still working on the VRD, which needs to be portable and cost-effective for people with low vision.

An electronic chip is also being developed that will rest on the nonfunctioning retina. The implanted chip will substitute for the retina, receiving light and electrically stimulating a layer of the retina's cells, creating visual images. The retinal implant system, which could be useful to people with macular degeneration and retinitis pigmentosa, consists of a camera and two microchips. A small electronic camera clipped on the user's eyeglasses will take in an image of the world. The first microchip sits on the glasses to send power and a laser image of the world to the second, or stimulator, chip, which rests on the retina, inside the eye. This chip will decode the sent image and transmit electric pulses to the cells in the retina. Researchers expect these pulses will be carried to the brain by the optic nerve and provide a useful image for the user.

A basic prototype of the implant system has already been developed and "proof of concept" experiments with animals have been performed. The next goal is to carry out short-term experiments with volunteers. The implant will probably not be ready to treat these diseases within the next five years, and the chip will surely be costly. The good news, though, is that the device might also be made to operate with other parts of the eye besides the retina. Many scientists in the United States and Germany are already working on electronic chips that hook up to the back of the retina, the optic nerve, and right on the visual cortex of the brain!

Scientists are developing other technologies to solve the problem of low vision. A technique called *adaptive optics* is revolutionizing both the diagnosis and the treatment of diseases in the back of the eye. Adaptive optics, first used by the military to sharpen images from telescopes, allows people to see at high resolution. It works by collecting light waves with a mirror and adjusting their shape to compensate for distortions in the image.

This technology can enhance images on a microscopic level, which means that when these adaptive optics instruments are available, doctors will be better able to see what is happening in the inner eye. Whether it is a doctor or a patient who is peering through an adaptive optics device, the world looks sharper. In tests of adaptive optics, people have declared a six-fold improvement in their sensitivity to contrast, being able to see fine stripe patterns that are indistinguishable even to people with 20/20 eyesight. Simply put, adaptive optics has the potential to make human eyes sharper than an eagle's!

Scientist David R. Williams of the University of Rochester in New York has already used adaptive optics to detect retinal diseases, and is attempting to use the technology to make glasses or contact lenses that correct for these diseases. He has constructed a special camera with a flexible mirror that he can use to identify and measure the distortions of the retina in a person with eye disease, and he believes that glasses or contacts using the same system could improve a person's vision by compensating for bumps and holes in the retina.

We can expect more and more of these extraordinary devices in the future. Still, we should not expect them to replace our human friends entirely, and we certainly cannot expect them to work right all the time. Anybody who has tried to set the timer on a VCR or keep a personal computer operating smoothly knows exactly just how exasperating these "timesavers" sometimes are. I recently had an experience that demonstrated just how unscientific and mysterious technology can be.

The Pitfalls of Too Much Technology

When daylight saving time came this spring, I discovered that setting all my clocks forward was an almost impossible task. I tried first with my digital bedside clock, pushing a series of buttons, but nothing happened, so I called a neighbor to help. He quickly reset the clock and my talking wristwatch.

About an hour after I had gone to bed that night, however, the alarm went off. I pushed what I thought was the "off" button, but minutes later the alarm rang again. I hit "off" *again,* but a few minutes later the alarm was sounding! I realized that when I had tried to set the time earlier in the day, I must have accidentally hit a button that set up the "snooze alarm" function. The only thing I could do was pull the plug!

By now I was so wide-awake that sleep was impossible. I got up and heated some milk. As I sat in the living room sipping my drink, I was startled by a synthesized woman's voice saying, "All is well." Whether this was my talking calculator or my talking watch, I will never know, but the message was vaguely reassuring.

Finally, I went back to bed, fell asleep, only to be wakened an hour or so later by Charlie announcing from the direction of my computer, "It is now safe to turn off your machine." While I was glad to hear it was now safe, I wondered why Charlie had chosen this particular time to make his pronouncement.

The next day I decided that my neighbor and I would check all my suddenly talkative helpers, and make sure all the clocks and controls were set to behave.

That night I foolishly looked forward to an uninterrupted night's sleep. But not long after I had drifted off, I heard a rooster crowing. Twelve times I heard him crow. I followed the barnyard racket to my talking wristwatch. In desperation I wrapped it in a shirt and stuffed it in a box that I threw in the back of the closet. That took care of the rooster for the rest of the night. Fortunately, I had been given another talking watch that I pressed into service the next day because I never did figure out how to get rid of the rooster. So every night at the same time I still hear that dim rooster crow from the corner of my closet, reminding me that technology is still a mysterious thing.

CAMEOS

 **Pam Jackson** is one of the vendors I was referred to when buying my personal computer. She gave me an opportunity to try out the equipment before I purchased it. Pam is now 35 years old and has had low vision from retinitis pigmentosa since she was a young child in Denver.

Because she had several brothers and sisters, she learned to read before attending school. According to the law then in effect in Colorado, she attended a special class for children with disabilities. This was upsetting because she knew more about reading than the other children.

A few years later her family moved to Montana where she could be in a regular classroom, and there she found she could keep up with the other children. Pam has always been a great lover of music, and in high school when she heard students were trying out for parts in the school musical, "The King and I," she begged for an audition. The director of the play did not know how to handle this. How could they have a "blind" child in the cast? But they were astonished at how well she sang, and she won the role of one of the king's wives. Each year after that Pam appeared in the school musical, and in her senior year she had the lead in "Hello Dolly."

After she moved to Seattle, Pam started working at the low-vision clinic of the Community Services for the Blind and became adept in using the JAWS software program. Later she heard that the company that created JAWS was looking for someone to represent them to visually disabled people, and she applied for the job. The owner of the company, Ed Henter, is blind himself, so he knew from experience that if people want to, they can surmount a visual disability. Pam won the account, and that was the beginning of her own company, Blink Soft Devices.

Today Pam represents several manufacturers of devices for the visually impaired and attends conferences for low-vision technology all over the country. She travels with Tempest, her seeing-eye dog, wherever she goes.

When she came to my apartment to give me a series of three hands-on demonstrations of JAWS, I confessed that having to master new key commands without a mouse or monitor was proving more difficult than I expected. But Pam told me the most important thing was determination—something I have heard over and over: "If you want to master new skills, you can."

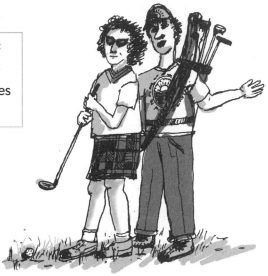

CHAPTER 11

Recreation Is Good for the Soul

A heart-shaped plaque with letters in wrought iron hangs on my living-room wall: "A Merry Heart Doeth Good Like a Medicine." I don't know when or where I acquired this simple treasure, but for years, wherever I have lived, it has found a place of prominence in my home. It speaks so clearly to my own sentiment.

Most of the time this "merry heart" can be brought about by a generally positive outlook on life, but sometimes it takes deliberate action to bring happiness and lift your spirits. Entertaining yourself—keeping busy with interesting activities both alone and with friends—can be a key to keeping close to the joy in life.

All Kinds of Music

In Chapter 7 I talked about music and the enormous influence it has had on my life. It calms me when I am agitated, I meditate to it, and sometimes I relax by dancing alone to my favorite string concerti or swing music. I regularly attend symphony concerts in the city and I have always loved to dance, whether in a public space or my own living room.

Concerts do not require vision, and they can be soothing or exciting. Plus, they are a great excuse to get together with friends and to go out on the town—feasting, listening to a wonderful concert, and talking about it afterward. In the summer, city parks often hold outdoor concerts that are either free or low-priced. These are opportunities to get together with others who have an interest in music.

Dance events of all kinds, from square dancing to ballroom dancing, are held in public spaces like senior centers and city festivals. The senior center near me even has hula dancing that anybody, young or old, can participate in. If you enjoy the younger scene, you can also find dance clubs in every city. Even totally blind people can participate in dancing, and it is a favorite pastime of many people I have talked with who have low-vision diseases. And, of course, it is great exercise.

Some people I know enjoy singing—either regularly in a church choir or with some other organized singing group, or on their own. If you are getting on in years, you could team up for a duet with someone else who remembers classic singers like Frank Sinatra and Bing Crosby. If you played an instrument in your youth, why not take it up again? Put yourself on a practice schedule just for fun, then perform for relatives or friends. A woman who attends meetings of my writers' group never passes up the opportunity to play the piano for us when one is available, which adds to the pleasure of our get-togethers.

A lot of literature in large print that is *about* music is distributed all over the world. The National Library Service for the Blind and Physically Handicapped (NLS) mails out thousands of sheet-music scores and books and magazines about music every year. I recently listened to a taped biography of Mozart by Marcia Davenport. Materials about music come in at least three formats: large-print, braille, and on cassette. The resources are free through each state's Talking Books Library, which is connected to the much larger National Library of Congress (see Chapter 5). The regional libraries distribute these items mostly to local people, but they will send a tape or a music score to other regions of the country if it is specifically requested.

Books That Talk

Two more kinds of entertainment will surely provide you with hours of intellectual stimulation. "Books on tape" and "talking books" are two forms of recorded literature.

Books on tape are commercially produced. They are refined in packaging—they might have a musical background and the narration is by professional actors. Books on tape are marketed to the person driving home from work and listening to the tape in the car, so often the versions are shorter than the original work—they have been abridged. It is more like listening to a radio or TV program. The local branch of your public library probably lends these out and carries a list of their books on tape. Your neighborhood video-rental store, such as Blockbuster Video, may rent them, and they are a big item in bookstores. Typical books on tape are the works of Stephen King, Agatha Christie, and Deepak Chopra.

The second kind of recorded literature is talking books. Even though they appear to be normal tapes, most talking books have *four* sides. This special NLS format allows extended recording time on a cassette tape and helps ensure that these free services are used only by people who truly need them. Only the first two sides can be played on a regular tape player; you need a special player to listen to sides three and four.

Talking books are distributed only through the Library of Congress and local Talking Books Libraries. The readers are sometimes actors, but usually they are simply people with good reading voices who volunteer. Talking books are usually unabridged and offer a large selection of topics—including romances, mysteries, history, biography, business, and specialized nonfiction.

The local Talking Books Library will send out a new catalog of selections every other month at no cost to people with low vision. (Your regular city library won't have these catalogs.) Talking books and the equipment to play them are sent postage-free directly from the NLS in Washington, D.C., on a three-month renewable loan. Anyone registered with a local talking books program can borrow the tapes. Call "Voices of Vision" at 202-707-5100 to register and order talking books. When returning these tapes by mail, you qualify for "Free Matter for the Blind"—all you have to do is flip the address card over so it is now addressed to the library from which it came. It will be picked up by the mail carrier and returned postpaid.

I was amazed at the number and variety of books on tape and talking books. The National Library Service circulates millions of titles every year through 57 regional libraries all around the nation. The Florida library is largest—it alone has a circulation of 2 million! Many people I have talked with across the country praise these tapes as one of their chief forms of entertainment.

You may find yourself interested in a book that isn't yet sold on tape in the stores or available through the Library of Congress. If you have a friend who likes to read, you might ask this friend to read a chapter at a time onto tape. When you are done with the tapes, give them to your favorite charity—surely at least one other person will enjoy hearing them too! You could also make your own audiobook with a tape recorder—record your memoirs and have a friend edit and copy them for your family and friends.

What's on the Radio?

The television has taken radio's place as the family's entertainment, but the radio can still be a wonderful source of amusement, especially for people who cannot see well. The variety of music available on the radio is better today than it was before television, providing country music, oldies, jazz and blues, even entire classical works and operas.

News and storytelling programs make their home on the radio, too, especially on National Public Radio. One of my favorites is Garrison Keillor's "Prairie Home Companion." Most public radio stations send out a schedule of their programs if you make a donation, small or large. If you cannot read the program, have a family member or friend go over it with you. Public-radio programming often includes readings from books, discussions of public affairs, weather forecasts, and sometimes dramatic programs.

People with low vision can tune in to more audio programming by turning their stereo televisions into radios. Books, magazine articles, and local and national newspapers are read by announcers and broadcast over the Radio Reading Service's "Second Audio Program" (SAP) channel, produced by WBGH radio in Boston. Public television stations in every major city in the United States carry at least one of these channels.

On the SAP channel, you can hear short stories on "The Western Hour," "The Science Fiction Hour," and "The Romance Hour." Old-time radio programs air regularly. Magazines, periodicals, and newspapers are read out loud, including the *Wall Street Journal,* the *Christian Science Monitor,* the *New York Times,* and *Rolling Stone* magazine, as well as local periodicals. The focus of the Radio Reading Service is "information of immediacy" such as newspapers, shopping ads, weekly magazines, and special news for those who cannot easily read printed material.

SAP programming transmits on a special frequency that is received only by stereo televisions. To tune in SAP programming, turn the channel selector to your local public television station and push the button on your TV or VCR remote control labeled "SAP," "MTS," or "Audio B." Your remote should have a button with one of these labels. If your TV or VCR doesn't bring in the SAP channel, call your public TV station—they provide special SAP radio receivers free of charge. If for some reason you cannot get a receiver from your public TV station, TV sets can also get SAP with a stereo audio receiver, sometimes called a decoder or adapter, which is available through Recoton. Don't pass up Second Audio Programs—you can enjoy many hours of listening pleasure with their diverse offerings.

Similar to Second Audio Program is Newsline for the Blind, an automated service developed by the National Federation for the Blind that reads newspapers over the telephone. By dialing a certain telephone number, you can listen to daily and Sunday editions of the *New York Times,* the *Chicago Tribune,* and *USA Today* for free. You don't have to be a member of the National Federation for the Blind—just call your local outlet for an access code. Dial the phone number for the Newsline, punch in the access code, and you can get the news every day without subscribing to a newspaper!

One warning, however. It would be best to own a speakerphone (a small speaker attached to the telephone that makes hands-free listening possible; many inexpensive telephones today have the feature built in) to listen to Newsline. Your hand will tire and your ear will ache if you are forced to hold a telephone receiver for an entire reading of the Sunday *New York Times*!

More Ways to Have Fun at Home

Now here are a few more good ideas for when you find yourself alone and wanting some fun.

• **Call your friends and relatives long distance for a conversation.** Surely you have some relatives or old friends in a far-off city who would love to hear your voice again. The best long-distance phone rates are in the evenings and weekends (or with some telephone companies, 24 hours a day), so take advantage of these times and have a nice hour-long conversation with someone you love.

• **Create simple parties for your friends and relatives** who live near you. This is for their sake as well as yours—everybody needs companionship. Don't worry about cooking for guests; order takeout or have food delivered. Potlucks or picnics are other ways to combine meals and fun. Or you could hold a tea party, which is easier than a full dinner. By all means, don't wait to be invited to a party and end up feeling sorry for yourself for being left out! Parties could include charades and other games, or just good conversation. Games with enlarged numbers and letters are available, including bingo, Scrabble, Monopoly, backgammon, and of course playing cards. You can buy all of these games through the low-vision catalogs listed in Resources. Remember, the idea is just to get people together and have fun.

• **"Descriptive Video Service" (DVS) on home video and television** offers audio-described movies for people who have low vision. As of this writing, hundreds of DVS titles are available for rental at video stores, including new releases, family and children's classics, comedy, drama, action adventure, science fiction, westerns, musicals, documentaries, and mystery classics. Free schedules of DVS programming on television are available through your local public TV station. If you have neighbors or friends who like movies, you can invite them over to watch these audio-described videos with you. Don't forget the popcorn!

- **Besides books on tape, many libraries also have old radio programs** available on cassette tape. You can listen to these by yourself or have others over to join in the fun and reminiscing.

- **Start a writing group.** Gather friends and write on a subject such as your most unforgettable experience, then (if you cannot read or do not wish to) have someone read each poem or essay out loud to the group. You don't have to have perfect vision to enjoy these kinds of activities.

Live Performances

To stay active, try to schedule regular trips out on the town. Attend poetry or book readings and lectures by inviting someone along who can drive, or use a van service or take the bus together. People with low vision can still enjoy the theater. One theater buff I know is a retired psychiatrist whose macular degeneration does not keep him away from the theater. He orders front row seats in advance so he can be sure to see and hear what's going on. Many theaters provide headphones to people with low vision that channel in a description of the action on stage. Before each show, patrons use a receiver (a device about the size of a small cassette tape player) to listen to descriptions of the main characters and samples of their voices, as well as a description of the set. During the show, a live narrator describes the events on stage as they happen.

I attended such a program to find out what they were like, and while I could hear nearly everything the actors said, I would have been confused if I hadn't heard the plot explained ahead of time and heard the action described as the actors spoke their parts. The narrator not only referred to the characters by name, but also described them in such a way that I could see what part they were playing in the drama. Audio described theater, I have heard, is now available in Great Britain, Japan, and Canada, as well as all over the United States, and a similar headset narration is now available at many movie theaters.

For Those Who Like to Travel

Many people with low vision still experience the world through travel. A surprising number of people I have talked with travel to new places, despite their vision.

Elderhostel programs for seniors that include lodging, activities, and tours have events all over the world. (See Resources for contact information.) Many cruise lines offer special cruises for people with low vision. "Eyes Only," a newsletter published by the Association for Macular Diseases, keeps tabs on some of these. Call QE Cruises at 212-988-4306 for more information, or ask your local travel agent.

People with macular degeneration can get a general impression of places they travel to both on cruises and land tours. We can see everything but the details—we can tour medieval churches, explore ancient palaces, see statuary, and get powerful impressions even of paintings. People with retinitis pigmentosa can see exquisite details in art or architecture even if they cannot take in cityscapes as well as they used to.

What I find most stimulating about foreign travel is immersing myself in a new culture. Although I can't understand the language, I find music in the tones of a foreign tongue. A great deal can be enjoyed about the people of another country just by mingling among them on the streets, on beaches, in restaurants, on trains, and at public attractions. And sometimes you have the greatest pleasure of all: to be invited into the home of someone you have met casually. All these experiences are possible, even with diminished vision.

If you yearn to travel and lack the funds, you don't have to leave our native shores to get a taste of foreign countries. Most cities have cultural festivals—Chinese, Mexican, Greek, Scandinavian—that are intended for everybody. Persuade someone to go with you, and observe the culture with all of your senses. Often part of the festivities will be ethnic dances, and food that will stimulate your sense of taste.

Developing Your Other Senses

Many partially sighted people develop greater auditory sensitivity, to compensate for the vision loss. In addition to hearing, focusing on your other senses is a good way to open up new avenues of entertainment.

The sense of touch

Petting zoos are designed with children in mind, but who's to say you can't enjoy them too? If there isn't a petting zoo nearby, see if you can get a personal tour of the animals at a regular zoo.

A docent at our zoo in Seattle told me about a woman who was completely blind. People kept telling her how large elephants are, so she asked if she could touch one. She was permitted to enter a cage with one of the keepers with a large, but gentle elephant. She was amazed as she stroked the animal's rough hide and touched its trunk and ears. But what astonished her most was that she could actually walk under this huge beast's belly—this, more than anything else, gave her a sense of how large an elephant is.

If you, too, would like to get closer to the animals, don't be afraid to ask. This is a wonderful way to permit your other senses to come to life. Though you probably have enough vision left to gauge the size of zoo animals and to see how they move about, you can use your hearing to be amused by their chatter and your sense of touch to experience how they feel. (Your sense of smell can come into play too, indicating just which animals you are near!)

The sense of taste

In addition to experiencing foods from different cultures at ethnic festivals, you can develop your sense of taste at home too. Host a dinner with an ethnic theme where guests bring dishes from a particular culture or mix it up and have food from many traditions. You could provide bread and beverages. Or have a tasting of a particular food. People who are into gardening have been known to have "tomato taste-offs" to see which variety tastes the best.

Olive oil (also the preferred oil; see Chapter 8) is another item that could be tasted. Use pieces of French bread to dip into different kinds and flavors of oil. (I have a fondness for this topic after spending 12 years as home economist for the Spanish Olive Oil Institute. I would also add that olive oil should not be kept in the refrigerator.) The history and culture of olive oil production is fascinating; perhaps someone could do some research for your party. Use your imagination and you can have all kinds of fun developing your sense of taste.

Sports, Believe It or Not

People who exercise live longer and are healthier in general. Sports have the double benefit of increasing circulation and getting you together with others to have fun. And having fun just might generate as many positive effects as anything else.

Golf is one sport that most people would assume those with low vision could not possibly join, but even completely blind people play golf. The United States Blind Golfers Association (USBGA) organizes golf tournaments for players who are blind. They publish a quarterly newsletter ("The Midnight Golfer"), and plan to release an instructional video for coaches and blind golfers. People with macular degeneration usually retain their peripheral vision, which is important in golf—and looking out for the sand traps and other hazards could be good exercise for your eyes. In fact, why not enter a competition? The USBGA tournament, the Ken Venturi Guiding Eyes Classic, is held every summer in Mount Kisco, New York. For more information about this club or its tournament, call 850-893-4511 or look up their site on the World Wide Web: www.igolf.com/organizations/usbga/index.htm.

Hiking is another activity that people with low vision can fully enjoy. In the Pacific Northwest, hiking clubs for the visually impaired offer the services of guides who accompany hikers. Going for a hike can be a great way to stimulate your other senses: listen to rustling leaves, feel the cool water of a mountain lake, smell the flowers, and taste the fresh air.

Similar organizations exist for skiers, and one can take lessons for developing the special skill of skiing with low vision. One group in my area teaches visually impaired adults how to cross-country ski, and the SKIFORALL foundation provides Nordic and alpine skiing and hiking instruction. This same foundation teaches water-skiing, river rafting, bicycling, and in-line skating to people with disabilities.

I have seen an association that offers one-day sails, sailing lessons, and other sailing opportunities to people who are visually impaired. For more than 20 years Disabled Sports USA has offered a variety of adaptive sports programs and events. Programs support each participant's ability to be active and independent, and include downhill skiing, kayaking and canoeing, soccer, and horseback riding. Disabled Sports USA also holds competitions and trains the instructors who teach the sports to others.

There are so many sports that are played by people with low vision, one begins to wonder: is there anything we can't do?

CAMEOS

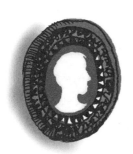

Jesse Minkert has been involved in artistic endeavors all his life. Jesse's own vision problem inspired him to found the Arts Access program for the visually impaired in Seattle. Now 50 years old, Jesse has had diabetic retinopathy for 15 years. Abnormal blood vessel growth on the surface of his retina blurs and interferes with his vision. Before he had trouble with his vision, Jesse earned a master's degree in sculpture, and was a painter and photographer. He had to give up painting a couple of years ago because of health problems caused by his diabetes and because his basement studio lacked sufficient lighting. Jesse also has talent as a writer of short stories, and when his vision was threatened he wrote and produced a radio drama.

Today, Jesse is involved in a number of projects, including audio description (live and tape-recorded) for theaters, art exhibitions, and dance performances. He and his wife Joan publish "Arts Access," a bimonthly publication that lists upcoming plays at local theaters that have audio description through headsets. They are recording or narrating training videos for businesses to show prospective low-vision employees. And they have designed a program for low-vision teenagers to learn to use audio equipment in a studio environment. Most of the teens are musicians who record and mix their own music with sound effects, but some also create dramatic plays for radio. Jesse feels his Arts Access projects are of special benefit to young people with vision problems because cultural education is not typically a priority for them. "Cultural access is easily neglected," he says.

Future projects include making available more discounted theater tickets and transportation vouchers for people with low vision. Cost and transportation are two major obstacles facing people with low vision who would like to attend cultural events. Another item on Jesse's wish list is to provide live narrations of big parades for visually impaired audiences.

Janai Fuller of Seattle got macular degeneration in one eye about seven years ago when she was 40 years old. What does Janai do for entertainment? She has played the violin her whole life, and when I spoke with her, she was soon to perform in a production of "Victor, Victoria." Janai also teaches music and sometimes records for movies as a freelance musician.

Janai's wet macular degeneration has stabilized: she sees well out of her right eye and has plenty of peripheral vision in her left eye. "The first few years, I kept coming up against my eyes. But you can't fight it. The only thing that'll happen is your blood pressure will rise. I didn't have a very good attitude at the beginning. Now I've adjusted—many times I don't think about it; now I just tune it out like the blurring is just not there." Because her vision has not deteriorated completely, she enjoys reading in her spare time and plays cards twice a week.

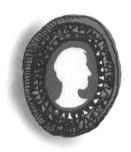

One of the advantages of living in a retirement community is the proximity to numerous helpers and others like you. My friend **Johannes Larsen** lives in a Fort Myers, Florida, retirement community where he is part of an activity group that includes 26 people who have macular degeneration. Some of these folks have joined a local support group specifically for visually impaired persons. The activities chairperson at the retirement community makes an effort to help residents with low vision continue activities they enjoy. For instance, they painted the shuffleboard disks white so players with macular degeneration can see them.

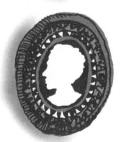

Two people in Johannes' support group are **Nina Giertsen** and **Phyllis Rutlin**. Nina likes to swim and plays a mean hand of bridge using super jumbo cards. First diagnosed with macular degeneration in 1983 at age 62, Nina says it has been fun finding ways to do those things that are undoable, like driving: "I drive a golf cart," she says. "You'll often hear a cry 'Be careful—here comes Nina!' But it only goes five miles an hour! I use my 'shank's mare,' too—my legs are still good." Phyllis loves to play the piano—this was her main hobby until being diagnosed with macular degeneration in 1995 at the age of 73. Though she cannot see the notes of sheet music anymore, her fingers know the keys. She can't read books or newspapers as easily now, but she loves large-print books and does large-print crossword puzzles.

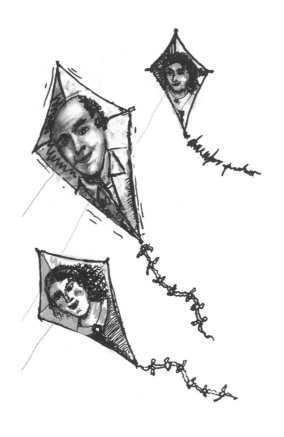

CHAPTER 12

Keep Your Spirits High and Your Kite Soaring

I have said it before and I will say it again because it is so important: the best treatment for low vision is a cheerful attitude. Look on the bright side. When you feel discouraged and depressed, think about how much better off you are than other unfortunate people you know, or visit a rehabilitation center for the disabled and watch people who are nearly or totally blind at work on difficult tasks. Then, swear to your inner soul, "If they can perform such difficult tasks, so can I!"

The cameos in this last chapter all reflect this spirit, and if this is not enough to convince you, let me quote a report from the Lighthouse in New York. They published the results of a study involving 150 people on the difference a positive attitude makes in adapting to vision loss. Five coping strategies were examined, and it was found that *optimism* had the single most positive effect on one's ability to adapt to vision loss.

Have you ever watched a kite soaring? It does not go bouncing off in the sky by itself. The person on the ground has to run with the kite until it catches a breeze, then must keep running and manipulating the string. That is what makes the long tail of the kite look so jaunty and proud. We need to work to keep the kite of our optimism soaring.

A Published Poet

The now-blind poet **Virginia Adair** is an example of the triumph of faith over anguish. When I told a friend about this book and my desire to talk with others who had lost their vision, she exclaimed, "You must talk with Virginia Adair. She lives in California, is totally blind, yet writes beautiful poetry. A book of her poems published by Random House has received much acclaim and there is talk of her being selected for the Pulitzer Prize."

I supposed her book might be about her blindness, so when I bought it I was puzzled by its strange title, *Ants on the Melon.* (She has since published another book, *Beliefs and Blasphemies.*) When I called her, I was even more astonished by her voice—a voice almost singing with the glow of life. It happened to be her eighty-sixth birthday.

Virginia told me that Helen Keller was actually a distant cousin of hers and, like Helen, she had attended Radcliffe College in Massachusetts. Virginia has overcome many difficulties in her life; her vision is just one of them. In addition to suffering the death of her husband, she has had multiple eye problems including cataracts, glaucoma, and an episode of bleeding in one eye that resulted in surgery to remove that eyeball entirely.

She's had eight ophthalmologists, one of whom would only see his patients "for four minutes, in and out." Another ophthalmologist's careless treatment was responsible for her glaucoma taking over. He was very rough, and when she pulled her head away to protect herself, he told her to leave his office if she couldn't hold still. None of her doctors were aware of the existence of the many low-vision clinics—Virginia actually heard about low-vision clinics and magnifiers by talking with the other people in her doctors' waiting room! Virginia has come to believe that a lot of doctors today are "drug pushers" in league with the big pharmaceutical companies, but she has finally found a woman doctor "who is an angel."

Most of her poems are exquisite pictures of scenes and emotions of times long past. In them, she recalls details of people and places full of meaning and beauty. It is clear that her vision loss alone is not the subject—that would be too narrow a focus; her feelings and memories are much more profound. Her pleasures and pains inspire her to keep going with her art.

A Delightful Farmer

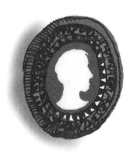

Just mentioning that I have macular degeneration to various people I run into frequently brings the response, "You should talk with my father—he has it too!" This was how I heard about **Don Wilson.**

I met Don Wilson's daughter at a meeting of my writer's club. When I explained that I hadn't been able to read the club's newsletter because of macular degeneration, she replied, "My dad has that! He's 77 years old and still drives the tractor around his farm."

She praised her father, telling me he was farming land that had been in their family since the time of the Revolutionary War. An ancestor of theirs, a Major John Wilson, was such a great military leader that the new American government, unable to give him money, instead granted him over 600 acres of land.

I called Don and discovered he was also hard of hearing—he thought I was a telemarketer trying to sell him something! As soon as I mentioned his daughter's name, his manner changed altogether and he told me with delight, "It's my birthday today!"

Don was diagnosed with macular degeneration a couple years earlier when he noticed that straight lines were turning crooked and the rows he was trying to work with his tractor were wavy. "My doctor wouldn't straight out tell me what was going on, though—he just said they didn't have any glasses strong enough to help me."

Since the death of his wife ten years ago, Don has lived alone, but he still has family that looks after him. His son lives right across the road and helps him around the farm, reads his mail to him, and gives him rides when he needs them. Don's granddaughter stops by every day on her way to school to drop off her little dog Chelsea for the day. He delighted in telling me that as soon as his granddaughter leaves for school, he looks at Chelsea and says, "Wanna go?" and she jumps in his truck.

He can see things in the distance pretty well, but he has to use a magnifying glass to read and write and he doesn't much bother with TV because he has to sit so close. When he is driving, he has difficulty seeing the different colors of the traffic lights in their little town, so he drives very slow, watching the drivers in front of him to see when they slow down.

Don enjoys the company of his family and working the ancestral farm. He raises 40 to 50 head of cattle, but says he's going to cut that in half so his son won't have to put out hay every day. He is slowing down a bit, but it's clear that not much can affect the spirit of this delightful personality.

A Farmer and a Traveler

 Coincidentally, around the same week I talked with another sturdy farm person: this time a woman, **Marie Waltz Farrell.** Her son Rich, whom I met at the low-vision support group, arranged for a three-way telephone conversation with Marie on her farm in Iowa.

Marie is 93 years old, and has had problematic vision all her life; despite this, she has maintained her farm home by herself, supervising a herd of 20 black Angus cattle since her husband's death 25 years ago.

Marie was just ten years old when she developed a cataract in her left eye, yet it was just four years ago that she had surgery to remove it. Her vision improved dramatically from the surgery—a few nights afterward she could see the wrinkles in her friends' faces. Then about a year later, her doctors detected signs of macular degeneration in the back of her eyes.

Before her husband died, he bought a farm adjoining theirs and rented it out; the renters pay Marie half of the profits from the sale of livestock as rent and look after her in a number of ways. She now hires someone to throw the hay out for the cattle. However, whenever a new bull is needed for the farm, she oversees its purchase, and at calving time she must be present because if something were to go wrong they could lose a calf very easily.

Despite her slipping vision, Marie drives on the backcountry roads and quilts and plays bingo down at her church—though she doesn't play as many cards as she used to; she used to play 18 cards at a time, but now she "only plays nine"!

I asked her if she still dreams of accomplishing something more in her life. "Oh, yes—I want to do a lot more traveling," she replied, and began listing the countries she had already visited. The first on the list was Liberia, West Africa, where one of her sons represents an American insurance company. After Liberia, she visited Rome, Greece, and Jerusalem, with other of her children, and spent six weeks in India with a granddaughter and her granddaughter's Japanese-American husband, who is an astronomer. Sometimes she tours with organized groups of farmers to visit the farms of other countries. Two of these were Russia and China, where the Chinese woman interpreter became her good friend and a couple years later brought her daughter to Marie's Iowa farm to visit. Marie keeps in touch with old friends, and her continued correspondence with a chum from grade school gave her an excuse to visit Australia. Marie said traveling to all those countries was a real education. "I never made it to high school," she said, "because I was the second oldest of 14 children, and I had to look after the younger kids."

It is wonderful that at 93 a person can have such a grand time keeping up the family farm, playing games, and traveling the world with her family. Marie seems to take her middle name literally—indeed, our conversation made me feel she is waltzing still.

A Publisher

Traveling through Brazil with the National Press Club group many years ago, I met **Ash Gerecht** and his wife Gloria, and we still keep in touch. Ash has had macular degeneration for three years, but

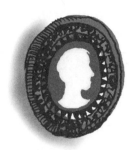

that hasn't stopped their touring. Just last year they went to Greece, and they plan to make other voyages but haven't decided just yet on their next destination.

Since Ash has one good eye, he is able to read and drive. For some 30 years he has been a publisher of newsletters. Ash goes to his office three times a week even though he has turned over the day-to-day business to his son. When we talked over the phone about the eye disease we share, he told me, "Some people get so frightened by the thought of losing their vision that they start worrying right away and it hinders their lifestyle. You have to accept what's happened, but continue to enjoy life."

A Photographer

Margret Prosser-Allan, a skilled artist and a passionate traveler, divides her time between her condo in Spain, her home in Delaware, and her family's homes in the Seattle area. One of the first memorable trips Margret took was to India—she accompanied her husband when he was sent there on a Fulbright scholarship. In fact, a book of photographs she took while there was displayed in an exhibition at the Smithsonian for several years.

After she became a member of the art department at the University of Delaware, Margret designed and built her own home. Then some years ago, at the age of 75, she developed macular degeneration (her older brother has it in a worse way). She can no longer paint or read normal print, but she continues to travel and take a lot of photographs.

She and her sister-in-law Mildred, known in the family as "Skip," are good friends. For the last few years, Margret and Skip have stopped in London on their way to Spain, and when they land they whiz through the airports in twin wheelchairs! Of Margret's instinct for art, Skip says, "We don't know how, but she still takes incredible photographs." Margret's nephew Dan confirms that she still appreciates color and texture, "and lives every day of her life like it's her first."

Still Working

 **Mary Hutchinson** was a lieutenant in the Navy's WAVES during World War II, and her husband was in U.S. Army intelligence. Mary was originally trained as an archaeologist—she has taken part in some important digs—and she and her husband continue to travel to a different country every year.

Even more meaningful to Mary is that they live in a hundred-year-old farmhouse in the District of Columbia, where the walls of every room are lined with books. Books are Mary's passion—she volunteers at the Salvation Army, sorting through the old donated books. At 86, Mary has dry macular degeneration and by now can barely read, but she carefully inspects each book with a magnifier to find the ones worth selling at the Salvation Army's popular annual book sale. Her extensive knowledge of authors and titles enables her to select the books worth restoring.

A Writer and Consultant

When **Sylvia Shur** was food editor of the *Woman's Home Companion,* I was on her staff. Later she became food editor at Parade, the

syndicated magazine section of many large city newspapers. When mutual friends told me Sylvia had macular degeneration, I phoned her in Westchester County, New York, to learn more. It was a delight to hear her voice after so many years, and I asked if I might include her cameo in my book.

"But I don't have macular degeneration," she said quickly. "It's another eye disease with a complicated name, uveitis. Some call it arthritis of the eye. It comes and goes, and I can still read a little and do a lot by touch." She said this nonchalantly, and I recalled this was typical of her offhand way of dealing with problems that might have others wheezing or wailing.

"And what are you doing now?" I asked.

"I'm still writing. I serve as a consultant to several food companies."

Of course! With her long career in the food field, a little thing like a vision problem would not stop her—touch, taste, and smell are just as necessary when questions about food arise. It did not surprise me at all to learn that Sylvia, always tiny and clever, was still on the job. Bless her.

Retired Actor Who Still Loves the Theater

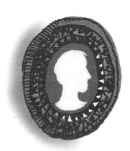

Paul Roland, 70, of Ashland, Oregon, is now retired from active stage life but receives residuals from films in which he appeared some years ago. He and his long-time companion, character actor Dee Maske, live in a restored house in this Oregon town famous for its devotion to Shakespearean theater. Paul's vision problems began with a detached retina some fifteen years ago. This led to damage to his macula. Now reading is difficult and his hearing is giving him problems. However, he still enjoys the theatrical life and accompanies Dee when she is offered out-of-town roles, including a role in Magic Fire at the Kennedy Center in Washington, D.C.

Keeping Her Family Together

Betty Cooper, who lives in Albuquerque, New Mexico, was first diagnosed with macular degeneration three years ago at age 56 when she went in for a regular eye exam. Today, she can read only large-print books for short periods of time, and says she misses reading magazines because most of the specialized ones she is interested in are not available in large print or on cassette.

Betty has found the love and support of her family to be the most fulfilling part of her life. She said her husband, who had polio as a child, has taught her to adapt and to see a way through anything. "You just have to believe," she said. Recently she started thinking of what she could do for someone else, so she became a "cuddler" for newborn babies at hospitals in Albuquerque. Betty's own six children are grown, and she and her husband are heading for retirement from their bookkeeping business.

As the psychiatrist Dr. Ladson Hinton observed, the eye is so dominant that any loss of vision can really make one feel cut off from the world, and at such times, we instinctively reach out for our families. Because Betty's children and grandchildren were scattered around geographically, she planned a seven-day cruise in the Caribbean, where they would enjoy a family reunion. The family had a wonderful time. Betty said it was a trip they will always remember: "It made us realize how much our family means to each of us and we all agreed to convene again in two years. The next time it will be in the Grand Cayman Islands in the Caribbean."

Sermons—and Cars

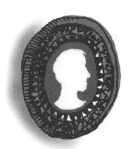

Several years ago, **Reverend James Arnold** was nearly blind due to cataracts in both eyes—he had 20/400 vision. When the cataracts were removed, he was astonished at how bright the world became—his visual acuity went to 20/30 overnight. But the clarity would not last forever: some years later Reverend Arnold became aware of another problem, and this time it turned out to be dry macular degeneration.

None of his vision problems have prevented him from keeping up his duties as pastor of his church, though. His knowledge of the Bible is so extensive that he is able to conjure up the basis of a sermon for every service. Reverend Arnold loves being with family, and his wife Joan is of tremendous assistance to him in his day-to-day activities. He is fortunate to have his children and grandchildren living within a few blocks of his home, and they check in on him regularly.

His main regret about vision impairment is that he can no longer drive. In memory of what fun it used to be to sit behind the wheel, he occasionally starts up his car in the garage and drives it down to the street and back again.

Writing His Memoirs

The assistance of others becomes all-important when one is living with low vision. Asking for help is something **Walter Ristow** has

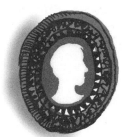

already learned to do. For many years, Walter served as chief of the map division at the New York Public Library and later at the Library of Congress. Walter retired in 1978, and moved to the Collington Life Care Community in Maryland in 1987.

In August 1996, Walter was stricken with macular degeneration, so he can no longer continue his passion for maps. Instead, he is writing his memoirs for his children and a regular editorial for the Collington newsletter. He is carrying on a campaign requesting the community's management to establish a structured program for the more than 50 residents who have low vision. Like so many of us, he uses a CCTV on a daily basis and relies upon a "seeing eye friend," a neighbor with whom he meets at least once a week to read mail, write checks, and visit doctors. Walter's son, who lives nearby, drove him around to find a big monitor for his personal computer, and adjusted the size of its letters for easier viewing.

Walter cannot always recognize people when they pass on the sidewalk, so he tries to get fellow residents to call out their names. In an article he wrote for the newsletter, he explains, "This will make our greetings more personal and I am asking that the rest of you follow this practice when you meet me or other low-vision residents. Thanks, and I will be Hearing You."

Other Ways of Seeing

When **Agnes (Aggie) Zinn** heard about the book I was writing, she called to ask my advice. People were advising her to move from her Seattle house into a retirement community, but she hated to leave her home. "Trouble is," she said, "I love gardening, but I can't see

 well enough to tell the weeds from the smaller flowers." She mentioned that she was quitting her garden club because it made her too upset not to be able to tell the differences among colors of flowers. I urged her not to give up her club, no matter what decision she might make about moving. I told her, "You need to get out and be with people!"

Recently, Aggie called me again. She wanted me to know she had sold her house and moved into a new retirement community and was so glad she had. "I've met so many interesting people here, and we have good times together," she said. "It is a relief not to have all those worries about the house and the yard." She added a comment that still echoes in my head: "You're going to be about as happy as you make up your mind to be."

• • •

It seems we all come to a time in our lives when we need to develop a new perspective on ourselves. This is true for everybody in the world, but especially true for those of us who have lost vision. We must replace that outer vision with an inner vision—a new way of seeing.

Resources

PART A

Organizations and Associations

AARP
See *American Association of Retired Persons*

Administration on Aging
U.S. Department of Health and Human Services
North Building, Room 4760
300 Independence Avenue SW
Washington, DC 20201
Phone: 202-245-0724
Emphasis: Develops and administers programs to promote the economic welfare and independence of older people and provides assistance to promote the development of state-administered, community-based social services for older people.

AFB Directory of Services for Blind and Visually Impaired Persons in the United States and Canada
See *American Foundation for the Blind (AFB)*.

AFB Press
American Foundation for the Blind
11 Penn Plaza, Suite 300
New York, NY 10001
Toll-free phone: 800-232-3044
Web site: www.afb.org
Emphasis: Develops, publishes, and sells informational books, pamphlets, periodicals, and videos for students, professionals, and researchers in

the blindness and visual-impairment fields.
See also *American Foundation for the Blind (AFB)*.

Against All Odds
See *Macular Degeneration Awareness*.

Aging and *Vision News*
Newsletters. See *Lighthouse, The*.

American Academy of Ophthalmology
P.O. Box 7424
San Francisco, CA 94120-7424
Phone: 415-561-8500
Fax: 415-561-8575
E-mail: member-services@aao.org
Web site: www.eyenet.org
Emphasis: Provides products, programs, materials, and services for
ophthalmologists, as well as referrals to local ophthalmologists; provides
fact sheets on visual impairments; sponsors the National Eye Care
Project; publishes a directory of medical and surgical eye care services
through the Committee for the Medically Underserved.

American Association of Retired Persons (AARP)
601 E Street NW
Washington, DC 20049
Phone: 202-434-2277
Emphasis: Provides assistance on legal issues, insurance, and a wide
variety of consumer products and other benefits; disseminates information on consumer affairs, health, financial, and disability issues; publishes *Modern Maturity* and *AARP Bulletin*.

American Association of the Deaf-Blind
814 Thayer Avenue
Silver Spring, MD 20919
Phone: 301-588-6545
Emphasis: Develops advocacy activities; holds annual convention for
deaf-blind people and their families.

American Bible Society

1865 Broadway
New York, NY 10023
Phone: 212-408-1200
Fax: 212-408-1512
Emphasis: Translates, publishes, and distributes biblical scriptures in braille, large-print, and recorded forms.

American Council of the Blind (ACB)

1155–15th Street NW, Suite 720
Washington, DC 20005
Toll-free phone: 800-424-8666 (3:00–5:30 P.M. EST)
Phone: 202-467-5081
E-mail: ncrabb@access.digex.net
Web site: www.acb.org
Emphasis: Provides referrals, legal assistance and representation, scholarships, consumer advocacy, and advice; promotes active participation by the blind in all aspects of society; distributes free monthly magazine (*The Braille Forum*) in multiple formats.

American Foundation for the Blind (AFB)

11 Penn Plaza, Suite 300
New York, NY 10001
Toll-free phone: 800-232-5463 (hotline)
Phone: 212-502-7600
TDD: 212-620-2158
NY residents: 212-620-2147
Web site: www.afb.org
Emphasis: Offers consultations for eye care rehabilitation through regional offices; serves as a national clearinghouse for information about blindness; publishes *AFB Directory of Services for Blind and Visually Impaired Persons in the US and Canada*; provides access to Careers and Technology Information Bank (CTIB) through the AFB National Technology Center.

American Macular Degeneration Foundation

P.O. Box 515
Northampton, MA 01061-0515

Toll-free phone: 888-MACULAR
Web site: www.macular.org
Emphasis: Works for the prevention, treatment, and cure of macular degeneration through raising funds, educating the public, and supporting scientific research. It is a 501(c)(3) nonprofit, publicly supported organization.

American Printing House for the Blind
1839 Frankfort Avenue
P.O. Box 6085
Louisville, KY 40206-0085
Toll-free phone: 800-223-1839
Phone: 502-895-2405
Fax: 502-899-2274
E-mail: aph@iglou.com
Emphasis: Provides textbooks for students who are visually impaired; maintains a centralized database of large-print, braille, and recorded books produced by the American Printing House, as well as materials from other publishers; provides free subscriptions to *Newsweek* and *Reader's Digest;* provides large-type textbooks, cookbooks, dictionaries, and the like; distributes free catalog and newsletters on cassette.

Arkenstone
555 Oakmead Parkway
Sunnyvale, CA 94086-4023
Toll-free phone: 800-444-4443
Phone: 408-328-8484
Emphasis: Sells computer software and scanners that translate printed material into simulated human speech.

Associated Services for the Blind
New Visions Store
919 Walnut Street
Philadelphia, PA 19107
Phone: 215-627-0600
Fax: 215-922-0692

Emphasis: Provides products for the visually impaired and produces periodicals in braille, tape, and large-print formats.

Association for Education and Rehabilitation of the Blind and Visually Impaired
206 North Washington Street, Suite 320
Alexandria, VA 22314
Phone: 703-548-1884
Emphasis: Promotes education and work for blind and visually impaired persons of all ages; conducts conferences; publishes newsletters and a journal; operates a reference information center; certifies rehabilitation teachers, specialists, and classroom teachers.

Association for Macular Diseases
210 East 64th Street
New York, NY 10021
Phone: 212-605-3719
Emphasis: Provides information for people with macular diseases; publishes a quarterly newsletter (*Eyes Only*); maintains a hotline for its members; conducts nationwide educational seminars on macular degeneration for the public.

Association of Radio Reading Services
WUSS Radio Reading Services
University of South Florida, WRB209
Tampa, FL 33620
Phone: 813-974-4193
Emphasis: Provides information on national radio reading services and broadcasts.

Audio Description
The Metropolitan Washington Ear
35 University Boulevard East
Silver Spring, MD 20901
Phone: 301-681-6636
Emphasis: Publishes a newsletter for individuals interested in audio description and provides information on national radio reading services.

Audio Editions
P.O. Box 6930
Auburn, CA 95604
Toll-free phone: 800-231-4261
Emphasis: Sells taped books for adults and children.

Audio Renaissance
Six Commerce Way
Arden, NC 28704
Toll-free phone: 800-452-5589
Emphasis: Sells taped books of popular fiction and nonfiction.

Bible Alliance
P.O. Box 621
Bradenton, FL 34206
Phone: 941-748-3031
Fax: 941-748-2625
Emphasis: Offers recorded biblical scriptures in 45 languages on cassette tapes free to the blind, visually impaired, and print-handicapped.

Blackstone Audio Books
P.O. Box 969
Ashland, OR 97520
Toll-free phone: 800-729-2665
Emphasis: Sells unabridged recordings of books.

Blindskills
P.O. Box 5181
Salem, OR 97304-0181
Toll-free phone: 800-860-4224
Phone: 503-581-4224
Fax: 503-581-0178
E-mail: blindskl@teteport.com
Emphasis: Publishes a quarterly magazine (*Dialogue*) in large print, braille, and four-track cassette tape designed for those who are experiencing vision loss.

Books on Tape
P.O. Box 7900
Newport Beach, CA 92658-7900
Toll-free phone: 800-626-3333
Fax: 714-548-6574
Web site: www.booksontape.com
Emphasis: Provides a library of full-length books to rent or purchase.
Also call your local library to rent books on tape.

Braille Circulating Library
2700 Stuart Avenue
Richmond, VA 23220-3305
Phone: 804-359-3743
Fax: 804-359-4777
Emphasis: Provides a library of books in braille, large-print, and talking
(audio) formats.

Braille Forum
Newsletter. See *American Council of the Blind (ACB).*

Braille Monitor
Newsletter. See *National Federation of the Blind (NFB).*

Careers and Technology Information Bank (CTIB)
See *American Foundation for the Blind (AFB).*

Carolyn's
1415–57th Avenue W
Bradenton, FL 34207
Toll-free phone: 800-648-2266 (9:00 A.M.–4:00 P.M. M–F EST)
Fax: 941-739-5503
Emphasis: Provides helpful products for the visually impaired,
ranging from talking calculators and thermometers to games and
TV enhancements.

CCLV News
Newsletter. See *Council of Citizens with Low Vision International (CCLV).*

Center for Self-Healing
1718 Taraval Street
San Francisco, CA 94116
Phone: 415-665-9574
Fax: 415-665-1318
Emphasis: Provides movement education and vision training.
See also *Schneider, Meir in Part B: Suggested Reading.*

Center for the Partially Sighted
720 Wilshire Boulevard, Suite 200
Santa Monica, CA 90401-1713
Phone: 310-458-3501
Fax: 310-458-8179
E-mail: lowvision@compuserve.com
Emphasis: Helps people of all ages with severe vision loss continue to
live, study, play, and work independently by providing comprehesive
vision rehabilitation programs. Optometrists who specialize in low-vision
design prescribe and fit individuals with optometric devices that maximize remaining sight. Rehabilitation specialists train people in daily living skills including safe and independent travel. Licensed clinical
therapists provide individual and group counseling of people with
severe vision loss and their families.

Chivers Audio Books
P.O. Box 1450
Hampton, NH 03843-1450
Toll-free phone: 800-621-0182
Emphasis: Sells taped books for adults and children.

Choice Magazine Listening
85 Channel Drive
Port Washington, NY 11050-2216
Phone: 516-883-8280
Fax: 516-944-6849
Emphasis: Offers free bimonthly anthology of unabridged articles, short
stories, and poetry from popular print magazines on four-track cassettes.

Committee for the Medically Underserved
See *American Academy of Ophthalmology.*

Community Services for the Blind and Partially Sighted (CSBPS)
(Washington state)
9709 Third Avenue NE, Suite 100
Seattle, WA 98115-2027
Toll-free phone: 800-458-4888
Phone: 206-525-5556 (voice/TDD)
Fax: 206-525-0422
E-mail: csbps@csbps.com
Web site: www.csbps.com
Emphasis: Offers rehabilitation and support services to visually impaired persons in Washington state; staffs an adaptive aids store and assistive technology center; offers volunteer assistance and educational services including information and referral; distributes free large-print newsletter (*Prism*) and free resource guide (*Visual Impairment and Blindness*).
Check your telephone directory for a similar service in your community.

Council of Citizens with Low Vision International (CCLV)
909 Southwest College Street
Topeka, KS 66606
Toll-free phone: 800-733-2258
Phone: 913-296-4454
Emphasis: Promotes the rights of visually impaired persons to maximize the use of their remaining vision; educates the public about the needs of visually impaired persons; publishes a newsletter (*CCLV News*); refers members to low-vision resources; grants scholarships to students majoring in low-vision rehabilitation.

Creative Adaptations for Learning (CAL)
E-mail: calinfo@cal-s.org
Web site: www.cal-s.org
Emphasis: Creates innovative tactile (embossed) illustrations to make pictures "visible" to blind children and adults, parents, teachers, therapists, and caregivers.

Delta Gamma Foundation
3250 Riverside Drive
P.O. Box 21397
Columbus, OH 43221
Phone: 614-481-8169
Emphasis: Provides services to blind and visually impaired persons through cooperation with local agencies.

Descriptive Video Service (DVS)
WGBH-TV
125 Western Avenue
Boston, MA 02134
Toll-free phone: 800-333-1203
Phone: 617-492-2777
Emphasis: Publishes a newsletter and provides information for individuals interested in descriptive video services.

Doubleday Large Print Home Library
Membership Services Center
6550 East 30th Street
P.O. Box 6325
Indianapolis, IN 46206
Toll-free phone: 800-321-7323
Phone: 317-541-8920
Emphasis: Provides hardcover editions of best-sellers in large print and on cassette; provides music tapes and videos.

Easier Ways
1049 Rock Hill Avenue
Baltimore, MD 21229
Phone: 410-644-4100
Fax: 410-644-4111
Emphasis: Offers consumer products for people who are blind or visually impaired.

Educational Tape Recording for the Blind
3915 West 103rd Street
Chicago, IL 60655
Phone: 312-445-3533
Emphasis: Offers recordings on cassette for students of all ages.

Eldercare Locator
Toll-free phone: 800-677-1116
Emphasis: Provides a nationwide referral service to help people find information about community providers of transportation, congregate and home-delivered meals, senior centers, and other services.
See also *National Association of Area Agencies on Aging.*

Elderhostels
Center for Studies of the Future
Phone: 805-648-6342
E-mail: ksb@elderweb.com
Web site: www.eldervision.org
Emphasis: Offers education and travel experiences for adventurous seniors.

Eye Bank Association of America
See *Lions Sight Conservation Foundation.*

Eyes Only
Newsletter. See *Association for Macular Diseases.*

Fighting Blindness News
Newsletter. See *Foundation Fighting Blindness, The.*

For My Patient: Macular Degeneration
Booklet. *See your local ophthalmologist for a copy.*
See also *Retina Research Fund.*

Foundation Fighting Blindness, The
Executive Plaza 1, Suite 800
11350 McCormick Road
Hunt Valley, MD 21031-1014
Toll-free phone: 888-394-3937

Phone: 410-785-1414
TDD Phone: 410-785-9687
Fax: 410-771-9470
Web site: www.blindness.org
Emphasis: Funds research to finding a cure and treatments for macular degeneration and related retinal degenerative diseases; publishes *Fighting Blindness News*; distributes free literature.

Foundation for Glaucoma Research
See *Glaucoma Research Foundation (GLF)*.

Foundation of the American Academy of Ophthalmology
See *National Eye Care Project™ (NECP)*.

Future Reflections
Newsletter. See *National Federation of the Blind (NFB)*.

G. K. Hall
See *Thorndike Press/G. K. Hall and Co.*

Glaucoma Research Foundation (GRF)
aka Foundation for Glaucoma Research
490 Post Street, Suite 830
San Francisco, CA 94102
Toll-free phone: 800-826-6693
Phone: 415-986-3162
Fax: 415-986-3763
E-mail: info@glaucoma.org
Web site: www.glaucoma.org
Emphasis: Sponsors and conducts research on glaucoma; provides comprehensive patient education materials and support services through the Glaucoma Support Network; publishes a quarterly newsletter (*Gleams*) and a patient guide (*Understanding and Living with Glaucoma*) which offers information about treatments and therapies and advice on coping with glaucoma.

Glaucoma Support Network
See *Glaucoma Research Foundation (GLF)*.

Helen Keller International
90 Washington Street, 15th Floor
New York, NY 10006
Phone: 212-934-0890
Web site: www.hki.org
Emphasis: Provides information on preventing blindness, restoring sight, and rehabilitation of the blind.

In Touch Networks
15 West 65th Street
New York, NY 10023
Toll-free phone: 800-456-3166
Phone: 212-769-6270
Emphasis: Maintains a volunteer reading service that reads articles from more than 100 newspapers and magazines via closed-circuit radio; makes referrals on similar services available in other areas.

Independent Living Aids (ILA)
27 East Mall
Plainview, NY 11803
Toll-free phone: 800-537-2118
Phone: 516-752-8080
Fax: 516-752-3135
Emphasis: Sells products designed for the visually impaired (as well as for those with arthritis and for the hearing impaired), including portable cassette players for talking books.

Institute for Families of Blind Children
Mail Stop #111
P.O. Box 54700
Los Angeles, CA 90054-0700
Phone: 213-669-4649
Emphasis: Publishes a free quarterly newsletter (*Parent to Parent*) for parents and professionals; offers counseling and support services in person or by telephone; provides resource books and tapes.

International Lions Club
300 22nd Street
Oak Brook, IL 60521
Phone: 630-571-5466
Emphasis: Provides free eyeglasses and exams; provides referrals for chapters and low-vision clinics in other areas.

Jewish Heritage for the Blind
1655 East 24th Street
Brooklyn, NY 11229
Fax: 718-338-0653
Emphasis: Offers free large-print Hebrew/English edition of *Yom Kippur Machzor* to the visually impaired.

John Milton Society for the Blind
475 Riverside Drive, Room 455
New York, NY 10015
Phone: 212-870-3336
Fax: 212-870-3229
Emphasis: Provides free religious and inspirational materials, including a quarterly magazine in large type, Bible study lessons in braille and on cassette tape, a braille magazine for youth (ages 8–18), and a directory of resources in large type.

Kurzweil
411 Waverly Oaks Road
Waltham, MA 02154
Phone: 617-893-5151
Emphasis: Sells personal readers that scan printed material and translate it into simulated human speech.

Library of Congress
National Library Service (NLS) for the Blind and Physically Handicapped
1291 Taylor Street NW
Washington, DC 20542
Toll-free phone: 800-424-8567
Phone: 202-707-5100

TDD phone: 202-707-0744
Fax: 202-707-0712
E-mail: nls@loc.gov
Web site: www.lcweb.loc.gov/nls
Emphasis: Conducts a national program that distributes free reading materials and recorded (talking) books and periodicals to individuals who have visual or physical impairments.
See Chapter 5 for details on this service.

Lighthouse, The
111 East 59th Street, 11th Floor
New York, NY 10022
Toll-free phone: 800-334-5497
Phone: 212-821-9200
TDD: 212-821-9713
E-mail: info@lighthouse.org
Web site: www.lighthouse.org
Emphasis: Distributes free consumer catalog of products designed to make life easier for the visually impaired; offers professional catalog of publications for doctors; offers help and hope to people of all ages through rehabilitation, education, research, and technical consultations; provides information, resources, education, printed materials, and consultations on visual impairment; sponsors the National Center for Vision and Aging and the National Center for Vision and Child Development; publishes quarterly newsletter (*Aging and Vision News*); provides information and referrals on low-vision centers and vision rehabilitation agencies in your locale.

Lions Club
See *International Lions Club.*

Lions Sight Conservation Foundation
Washington–Northern Idaho LSCF
901 Boren Avenue, Suite 810
Seattle, WA 98104-3508
Phone: 206-682-8500

Fax: 206-682-8504
Emphasis: Sponsors the Lions Eye Bank (through the Eye Bank Association of America); provides funds through patient-care grants; provides equipment and education through low-vision clinics; sponsors a mobile medical unit which offers free eye screening in communities across the country.

Listening Library
One Park Avenue
Old Greenwich, CT 06870-1727
Toll-free phone: 800-243-4504
Emphasis: Sells taped books for adults and children.

Love Bike, The
P.O. Box 1438
Boyes Hot Springs, CA 95416
Phone: 707-938-2429
Fax: 707-938-2459
E-mail: andy@lovebike.com
Web site: www.lovebike.com
Emphasis: Sells a tandem bike that can be used by children and the vision impaired.

Low-Vision Support Groups
Seattle, Washington
Phone: 206-461-7841 or 206-230-0166 for groups facilitated by Carin Mack, MSW
See also *Community Services for the Blind and Partially Sighted (CSBPS); International Lions Club; Lighthouse, The; and Macular Degeneration Awareness.*

LS&S Group
P.O. Box 673
Northbrook, IL 60065
Toll-free phone: 800-468-4789 (orders)
Toll-free TTY: 800-317-8533
Phone: 847-498-9777 (information and customer service)

Fax: 847-498-1482 (24 hours/day)
E-mail: lssgrp@aol.com
Web site: www.lssgroup.com
Emphasis: Sells products especially designed for the visual and hearing impaired, including computer adaptive devices.

Macular Degeneration Awareness
Against All Odds
c/o Morton Bond
700 S. Hollybrook Drive, #210
Pembroke Pines, FL 33025
Phone: 954-431-3111
Emphasis: Offers information and education on macular degeneration and conducts a support group.

Macular Degeneration Foundation
P.O. Box 9752
San Jose, CA 95157-9752
Toll-free phone: 888-633-3937
Phone: 408-260-1335
Fax: 408-260-1336
E-mail: eyesight@eyesight.org
Web site: www.eyesight.org
Emphasis: Conducts research and provides information regarding prevention and cure of macular degeneration; offers free (large-print) publication (*The Magnifier*) available via mail or the internet.

Macular Degeneration International
2968 West Ina Road, #106
Tucson, AZ 85741
Toll-free phone: 800-393-7634
Phone: 520-797-2525
Web site: www.maculardegeneration.org
Emphasis: Publishes *Around the Edges,* a bi-annual news journal that provides updates on medical and technological research, including vitamins; publishes direct mailings to members regarding local seminars and other items of interest.

Magnifier, The
Newsletter. See *Macular Degeneration Foundation.*

Massachusetts Association for the Blind
200 Ivy Street
Brookline, MA 02146
Toll-free phone: 800-682-9200 (MA only)
Phone: 617-738-5110
Fax: 617-738-1247
Emphasis: Offers consumer products for people who are blind or visually impaired.

Matilda Ziegler Magazine for the Blind
20 West 17th Street
New York, NY 10011
Phone: 212-242-0263
Emphasis: Offers free monthly general-interest periodical in braille and on disk.

Maxi-Aids
42 Executive Boulevard
Farmingdale, NY 11735
Toll-free phone: 800-522-6294
Fax: 516-752-0689
TTY: 516-752-0738
E-mail: sales@maxiaids.com
Web site: www.maxiaids.com
Emphasis: Sells products designed especially for the visually impaired, blind, hard-of-hearing, deaf, deaf-blind, arthritic, and physically challenged.

Microsoft Guide to Windows 95 Keyboard Commands
BRL, Inc.
Phone: 800-407-5839
E-mail: brlinc@mindspring.com
Emphasis: Offers tips for navigating Windows95 with keyboard strokes.

National Association for Parents of the Visually Impaired
Toll-free phone: 800-562-6265
Phone: 617-972-7441
Fax: 617-972-7444
Emphasis: Provides support to parents of children with visual impairments.

National Association for Visually Handicapped (NAVH)

New York:
22 W. 21st Street
New York, NY 1001
Phone: 212-889-3141
Fax: 212-727-2931
E-mail: staff@navh.org
Web site: www.navh.org

California:
3201 Balboa Street
San Francisco, CA 94121
Phone: 415-221-3201
Fax: 415-221-8754

Emphasis: Serves as a clearinghouse for information about services for those with visual impairment; serves as the "spokes-organization" for the partially seeing; conducts bicoastal community self-help groups; counsels in the testing and use of visual devices; sponsors professional and public educational outreach; provides referrals; conducts a large-print loan library by mail of over 6,500 titles; publishes a newsletter and large-print catalog (*Visual Aids and Informational Materials*).

National Association of Area Agencies on Aging
1112–16th Street NW, Suite 100
Washington, DC 20036
Phone: 202-296-8130
Emphasis: Operates Eldercare, which provides referrals for community services.

National Coalition for Deaf-Blindness
c/o Perkins School for the Blind
175 North Beacon Street
Watertown, MA 02172
Phone: 617-924-3434
Emphasis: Advocates for deaf-blind persons.

National Eye Care Project™ (NECP)
Foundation of the American Academy of Ophthalmology
P.O. Box 429098
San Francisco, CA 94142-9098
Toll-free phone: 800-222-3937
Emphasis: Provides access to no-cost medical eye care to qualified patients age 65 and over.

National Eye Institute
Information Center
Building 21, Room 6A32
31 Center Dr., MSC 2510
Bethesda, MD 20892-2510
Phone: 301-496-5248
Fax: 301-402-1065
E-mail: 2020@nei.nih.gov
Web site: www.nei.nih.gov
Emphasis: Conducts and funds research on eye and visual disorders and publishes materials on visual impairment.

National Federation of the Blind (NFB)
1800 Johnson Street
Baltimore, MA 21230
Phone: 410-659-9314
Fax: 410-685-5653
Web site: www.nfb.org
Emphasis: Offers national magazine and extensive literature in print and braille and on cassette; maintains referral and job services; publishes *The Braille Monitor* and *Future Reflections*; offers *Newsline for the Blind,* a newspaper service by telephone (to limited areas).

National Federation of the Blind of Washington
P.O. Box 2516
Seattle, WA 98111
Phone: 425-823-6380
Emphasis: Provides regional and national information and referrals

regarding services for the blind and visually impaired; sponsors "miniconventions" and conferences about ways blind and visually impaired people can succeed in their employment and social, civic, and family life.

National Library Service (NLS) for the Blind and Physically Handicapped
See *Library of Congress.*

National Resource Guide
See *Community Services for the Blind and Partially Sighted (CSBPS).*

National Retinitis Pigmentosa Foundation
See *RP Foundation Fighting Blindness.*

National Society to Prevent Blindness
See *Prevent Blindness America.*

New Visions Store
See *Associated Services for the Blind.*

New York Times
Large-type weekly newspaper
229 W. 43rd Street
New York, NY 10036
Toll-free phone: 800-631-2580
Phone: 212-556-1734
Fax: 212-556-1748
Emphasis: Offers subscriptions for home or business delivery of a large-print edition of the *New York Times.*

Newsline for the Blind
Newspaper by phone. See *National Federation of the Blind (NFB).*

Newspapers for the Blind
5508 Calkins Road
Flint, MI 48532
Phone: 313-230-8866
Emphasis: Provides telephone service of reading local newspapers over

the telephone to subscribers and provides information on services in other areas.

Nostalgia Television
3575 Cahuenga Boulevard, Suite 495
Los Angeles, CA 90068
Phone: 213-850-3000
Emphasis: Provides narration of key visual elements and action for many television programs and videos.

Perkins School for the Blind
See *National Coalition for Deaf-Blindness.*

Prevent Blindness America
(formerly known as National Society to Prevent Blindness)
500 East Remington Road
Schaumberg, IL 60173
Toll-free phone: 800-331-2020
Phone: 847-843-2020
E-mail: info@preventblindness.org
Web site: www.prevent-blindness.org
Emphasis: Provides information on vision, eye health and safety, research, and some community services; publishes *Prevent Blindness News* and *Wise Owl News.*

Prism
Newsletter. See *Community Services for the Blind and Partially Sighted (CSBPS).*

Reader's Digest
Large-type editions
P.O. Box 241
Mount Morris, IL 61054
Toll-free phone: 800-877-5293
Emphasis: Offers subscription to *Reader's Digest* and condensed books in large-print editions.
See also *American Printing House for the Blind.*

Reading Services
See *In Touch Networks.*

Recorded Books
270 Skip Jack Road
Prince Frederick, MD 20678
Toll-free phone: 800-628-1304
Emphasis: Sells best-sellers and classics in audio format.

Recorded Periodicals
See *Associated Services for the Blind.*

Recording for the Blind
The Anne T. MacDonald Center
20 Roszel Road
Princeton, NJ 08540
Toll-free phone: 800-221-4792
Phone: 609-452-0606
Fax: 609-987-8116
Web site: www.rfbd.org
Emphasis: Lends tape-recorded textbooks and other educational materials at no charge to visually, perceptually, and physically impaired students and professionals.

Resources for Rehabilitation
33 Bedford Street, Suite 19A
Lexington, MA 02173
Phone: 617-862-6455
Fax: 617-861-7517
Emphasis: Publishes large-print directories such as *Living with Low Vision: A Resource Guide for People with Sight Loss* and *Resources for Elders with Disabilities,* as well as large-print resource lists.

Retina Research Fund
P.O. Box 640350
San Francisco, CA 94164
Emphasis: Conducts research; publishes *For My Patient: Macular Degeneration.*

Retinitis Pigmentosa Foundation
See *RP Foundation Fighting Blindness.*

RP Foundation Fighting Blindness
National Retinitis Pigmentosa Foundation
1401 Mt. Royal Avenue
Baltimore, MD 21217
Phone: 301-225-9400
Emphasis: Conducts public education programs and supports research related to the cause, prevention, and treatment of RP; maintains a national network of affiliates; conducts workshops; conducts referral and donor programs.

Schepens Eye Research Institute
(originally known as the Retina Foundation)
20 Stanford Street
Boston, MA 02114
Phone: 617-912-0100
E-mail: geninfo@vision.eri.harvard.edu
Emphasis: Provides information on current eye research, concentrating on the causes and prevention of blinding eye diseases.

Social Security Administration
U.S. Department of Health and Human Services
6401 Security Boulevard
Baltimore, MD 21235
Phone: 301-965-1234
Emphasis: Oversees old age, survivors, and disability insurance programs, including Supplemental Security Income (SSI) program for aged, blind, and disabled persons; maintains a network of offices across the country and publishes a variety of materials on social security benefits.

Spectrum
The Lighthouse Store
111 East 59th Street
New York, NY 10022
Phone: 212-821-9384

Emphasis: Displays and sells a wide range of non-optical devices for people with impaired vision.
See also *Lighthouse, The.*

State Department of Services for the Blind
(Washington state)
Toll-free phone: 800-552-7103
Emphasis: Offers services to increase the independence, employment potential, and quality of life for blind and visually impaired persons statewide, including a vocational rehabilitation program, a residential orientation and training center, an independent-living program, child and family program, a business enterprise program, and an assistive technology center.
Check the government section or blue pages of your telephone directory for your state services.

State Rehabilitation Agency
(Washington state)
P.O. Box 45340
Olympia, WA 98504-5340
Toll-free phone: 800-637-5627
Emphasis: Provides assistance and rehabilitation services to people who are visually impaired.
Check the government section or blue pages of your telephone directory for your state services.

State School for the Blind
(Washington state)
2214 E. 13th Street
Vancouver, WA 98661
Phone: 360-696-6321
Emphasis: Provides specialized educational services to visually impaired and blind youth up to age 21 who are residents of Washington; serves as a statewide demonstration and resource center, and a technology support service for school districts.
Check the government section or blue pages of your telephone directory for your state services.

Talking Books
See *Library of Congress*.

Taping for the Blind
3935 Essex Lane
Houston, TX 77027
Phone: 713-622-2767
Emphasis: Provides recorded reading materials on cassette for use by visually and physically impaired persons.

Telesensory
520 Almanor Avenue
Sunnyvale, CA 94086-3533
Toll-free phone: 800-804-8004
Phone: 408-616-8700
Fax: 408-616-8719
Washington state phone: 425-401-5036
Web site: www.telesensory.com
Emphasis: Sells products designed to increase the independence of people with low vision, including talking CCTVs, computer magnification systems, reading software, and internet browsers.

Thorndike Press/G. K. Hall and Co.
P.O. Box 159
Thorndike, ME 04986
Toll-free phone: 800-223-6121
Phone: 207-948-2962
Fax: 800-558-4676 (toll-free)
Web site: www.yp.com/mlr/thorndike/index.html
Emphasis: Provides direct sale of large-print books.

VISION Foundation
818 Mt. Auburn St.
Watertown, MA 02172
Toll-free phone: 800-852-3029 (MA only)
Phone: 617-926-4232
Fax: 617-926-1412

Emphasis: Publishes the VISION Resource List, available in large print or cassette, containing a wide variety of free resources for the visually impaired.

Vision Rehab Centers
6343 West 95th Street
Oak Lawn, IL 60453
Toll-free phone: 888-744-4897
Phone: 708-952-3505
E-mail: llipschultz@visionrehab.com
Web site: www.vision.rehab.com
Emphasis: Provides low-vision care and devices at centers and clinics nationwide.

VISIONS/Services for the Blind and Visually Impaired
120 Wall Street, 16th Floor
New York, NY 10005-3914
Phone: 212-425-2255
Fax: 212-425- 7114
Emphasis: Offers free services to anyone over 55 with vision problems, including self-help study kits, rehabilitation training in the home, and year-round vacation camp for blind adults and their families.

Visual Aids and Informational Materials
See *National Association for the Visually Handicapped (NAVH).*

Visual Impairment and Blindness: A Resource Guide
See *Community Services for the Blind and Partially Sighted (CSBPS).*

Vocational Rehabilitation
See *State Rehabilitation Agency.*

Washington Assistive Technology Alliance
(Washington state)
606 West Sharp Avenue
Spokane, WA 99201
Phone: 800-214-8731
Web site: www.wata.org

Emphasis: Provides referrals for funding and sources for assistive technology.

World at Large
1689 46th Street
Brooklyn, NY 11204
Toll-free phone: 888-285-2743 (except in NYC)
Phone: 718-972-4000
Fax: 718-972-9400
Emphasis: Provides a biweekly large-print newspaper, including articles from magazines such as *U.S. News and World Report, Time,* and *The Monitor.*

Xavier Society for the Blind
154 East 23rd Street
New York, NY 10010
Toll-free phone: 800-637-9193
Phone: 212-473-7800
Emphasis: Produces religious and inspirational material in braille and large print and on tape.

Xerox Imaging Systems
Nine Centennial Park Drive
Peabody, MA 01960
Toll-free phone: 800-421-7323
Phone: 508-977-2000
Emphasis: Sells personal readers that scan printed material and translate it into simulated human speech.

PART B

Suggested Reading

Adair, Virginia Hamilton
Ants on the Melon: A Collection of Poems, New York: Random House, 1996.
Beliefs and Blasphemies, New York: Random House, 1998.

Alliance for Technology Access
Computer Resources for People with Disabilities, Alameda, CA: Hunter
House Publishers, 1996.

Bailey, Ian, and Amanda Hall
Visual Impairment: An Overview, New York: AFB Press, 1990.

Buckland, Clare
Always Becoming: An Autobiography, Vancouver, BC: Peanut Butter Press,
1996.

Dickman, Irving R.
Making Life More Livable, New York: AFB Press, 1991.

Goodrich, Janet
Natural Vision Improvement, Berkeley, CA: Celestial Arts, 1985.

Griffin-Shirley, Nora, and Gerda Groff
*Prescriptions for Independence: Working with Older People Who Are
Visually Impaired,* New York: AFB Press, 1993.

Hull, John
Touching the Rock: An Experience of Blindness, New York: Pantheon
Books, 1990.

Keller, Helen
Light in My Darkness (with Ray Silverman), revised edition, New York:
Swedenborg Foundation, 1995.

Midstream: My Later Life, New York: Greenwood Press, 1968.
Story of My Life, Thorndike, ME: G. K. Hall, 1993.

Levner, Henrietta
I Keep Five Pairs of Glasses in a Flower Pot, New York: National Association for the Visually Handicapped, 1985.

Ludwig, Irene; Lynne Luxton; and Marie Attmore
Creative Recreation for Blind and Visually Impaired Adults, New York: AFB Press, 1988.

Neer, Frances Lief
Dancing in the Dark: A Guide to Living with Blindness and Visual Impairment, San Francisco, CA: Wildstar Publishers, 1994.

Ringgold, Nicolette Pernot
Out of the Corner of My Eye: Living with Vision Loss in Later Life, New York: AFB Press, 1991.

Ross, Mary Alice
Fitness for the Aging Adult with Visual Impairment, New York: AFB Press, 1984.

Schneider, Meir, PhD, LMT
Miracle Eyesight Method (audiocassette), Boulder, CO: Sounds True, 1996.
Self-Healing: My Life and Vision, New York: Viking Press, 1989.
The Handbook of Self-Healing (with Maureen Larkin), New York: Penguin Books, 1994.

Weil, Andrew, MD
Eight Weeks to Optimum Health: A Proven Program for Taking Full Advantage of Your Body's Natural Healing Power, New York: Alfred A. Knopf, 1997.

Quick Guide to Internet Resources

Ability
Web site: www.ability.org.uk
Emphasis: Provides directory and links to resources related to general health and disability topics.

Achoo
Web site: www.achoo.com
Emphasis: Provides directory to healthcare news.

Age of Reason
Web site: www.ageofreason.com
Emphasis: Provides internet resource center and links to other sites of interest to the over-50 age group.

American Academy of Allergy, Asthma and Immunology
Web site: www.aaaai.org
Emphasis: Provides patient referrals, and public and professional information on health-related issues.

American Academy of Ophthalmology
Web site: www.eyenet.org
Emphasis: Provides information on health issues related to the eyes; provides referrals to local ophthalmologists.

American Council of the Blind
Web site: www.acb.org
Emphasis: Provides general information on activities on the council, access to monthly radio program (ACB Reports), and a monthly publication (*Braille Forum*).

American Foundation for the Blind
Web site: www.afb.org

Emphasis: Serves as a national clearinghouse for information about blindness.

American Medical Association
Web site: www.ama-assn.org
Emphasis: Provides information on health-related issues.

Ask Dr. Weil
Web site: cgi.pathfinder.com/drweil/
Emphasis: Provides information on alternative medicine from Dr. Andrew Weil.

Blind Net
Web site: www.blind.net
Emphasis: Provides information and links to resources for the blind.

BLINDAD
Computerized administrator: listserv@maelstrom.stjohns.edu
Human administrator: blindad-request@maelstrom.stjohns.edu
Emphasis: Welcomes blindness-related advertisements (personal and some commercial) and discussions of aids for partially sighted and blind people.
To subscribe: Send e-mail to the computerized administrator. In the body of the message, type: sub BLINDAD [your name or the name you want to be known by on the list].

Blind-Related Resources on the Internet
Web site: www.redwhiteandblue.org/blindmenu.html
Emphasis: Provides links to resources and services for the blind.

Blindness Resource Center
Web site: www.nyise.org/blind.htm
Emphasis: Provides information from the New York Institute for Special Education.

Blindness-Related Emailing Lists
Web site: www.hicom.net/~oedipus/blist.html
Emphasis: Provides comprehensive index of blindness-related e-mailing lists and newsgroups.

Books on Tape
Web site: www.booksontape.com
Emphasis: Provides a library of full-length books to rent or purchase.

Chocolate Braille
Web site: www.chocobraille.com
Emphasis: Sells chocolate braille greeting cards, guide dogs, and other novelties and gift baskets.

Community Services for the Blind and Partially Sighted (CSBPS)
Web site: www.csbps.com
Emphasis: Offers information about CSBPS programs and services.

Digital Journal of Ophthalmology
Massachusetts Eye and Ear Infirmary
Web site: www.djo.harvard.edu/
Emphasis: Provides information on research to prevent blindness.

DoctorNet
Web site: www.doctornet.com
Emphasis: Provides a comprehensive reference to medical information.

Eldercare Web
Web site: www.elderweb.com
Emphasis: Provides age-related resources.

Elderhostels
Center for Studies of the Future
Web site: www.eldervision.org
Emphasis: Offers education and travel experiences for adventurous seniors.

Eyecare
New Jersey Optometric Association
Web site: www.eyecare.org/
Emphasis: Provides information on eyecare and eyewear for consumers, as well as doctor referrals.

Focus
Web site: www.focusnewsletter.org

Emphasis: Provides an information forum for research and studies on retinal degenerative disorders, including alternative treatments.

Foundation Fighting Blindness
Web site: www.blindness.org
Emphasis: Provides information on research to find cures and treatments for macular degeneration and related retinal degenerative diseases.

Glaucoma Research Foundation (GRF)
Web site: www.glaucoma.org
Emphasis: Sponsors and conducts research on glaucoma; provides comprehensive patient education materials and support services; publishes a quarterly newsletter and patient guide that offer information about treatments and therapies, and advice on coping with glaucoma.

Glaucoma—What Is Glaucoma?
Web site no longer current
Emphasis: Provides information on glaucoma and links to other vision-related sites.

Glickman, Gary, MD, PC
Diseases and Surgery of the Retina
Web site: www.panix.com/~glickman
Emphasis: Provides information on diseases of the retina, including macular degeneration, and offers links to related sites.

Hardin Meta Directory of Internet Health Sources
Hardin Library for the Health Sciences, University of Iowa Libraries
Web site: www.lib.uiowa.edu/hardin/md
Emphasis: Provides directory of health-related resources.

Health WWWeb
Web site: www.teleport.com/~amrta/iwaywww.html
Emphasis: Provides links to medical and healthcare related sites.

HealthGate
Web site: www.healthgate.com
Emphasis: Provides information on health-related issues.

Healthlinks.net
Web site: www.healthlinks.net
Emphasis: Provides information and links for professional-level health-care resources.

Healthtouch Online for Better Health
Web site: www.healthtouch.com
Emphasis: Provides information and links for health-related resources.

Helen Keller International
Web site: www.hki.org
Emphasis: Provides information on preventing blindness, restoring sight, and rehabilitation of the blind.

Idealist
Action Without Borders
Web site: www.idealist.org
Emphasis: Provides information and links to over 14,000 organizations that help build a world where all people can live free, dignified, and productive lives.

Library of Congress
National Library Service (NLS) for the Blind and Physically Handicapped
Web site: www.lcweb.loc.gov/nls
Emphasis: Conducts a national program that distributes free reading materials and recorded (talking) books and periodicals to individuals who have visual or physical impairments.

Lighthouse, The
Web site: www.lighthouse.org
Emphasis: Provides information, resources, education, printed materials, and consultations on visual impairment; provides information and referrals on low-vision centers and vision rehabilitation agencies in your locale.

Love Bike
Web site: www.lovebike.com
Emphasis: Sells a tandem bike that can be used by children and the vision impaired.

Low Vision Discussion List

Computerized administrator: listserv@maelstrom.stjohns.edu
Human administrator: lowvis-request@maelstrom.stjohns.edu
Web site: tile.net/listserve/lowvis.html
Emphasis: Provides discussion group for professionals in clinical low-vision rehabilitation to interact with professionals in adaptive technology.
To subscribe: Send e-mail to the computerized administrator. In the body of the message, type: sub LOWVIS [your name or the name you want to be known by on the list].

Macular Degeneration Foundation

Web site: www.eyesight.org
Emphasis: Publishes online large-font newsletter (*The Magnifier*); provides reports on the latest research, requests for research participants, links, bulletin board, answers to frequently asked questions, list of low-vision centers and specialists, and an eye test.

Macular Degeneration International

Web site: www.maculardegeneration.org
Emphasis: Provides information on the organization's activities as well as information on current medical research on macular degeneration (large-font viewing available).

Macular Degeneration List

Computerized administrator: listserv@listserv.aol.com
Human administrator: MDList@listserv.aol.com
Emphasis: Provides a place to exchange helpful tips, experiences, and mutual encouragement among those experiencing macular degeneration.
To subscribe: Send e-mail to the computerized administrator. In the body of the message, type: SUB MDLIST [your name or the name you want to be known by on the list].

Massachusetts Eye and Ear Infirmary

Web site: www.meei.harvard.edu/meei
Emphasis: Provides information in affiliation with the Harvard Medical School related to disorders of the eye, ear, nose, throat, head, and neck; publishes the *Digital Journal of Ophthalmology*, a journal of research to prevent blindness.

National Association for Visually Handicapped (NAVH)

Web site: www.navh.org

Emphasis: Serves as a clearinghouse for information about services for those with visual impairment. The web site has a visual aids store, links, frequently asked questions, an e-mail discussion list, and a quarterly large-print newsletter.

National Eye Institute

National Institutes of Health

Web site: www.nei.nih.gov

Emphasis: Provides information on eye and visual disorders.

National Federation of the Blind (NFB)

Web site: www.nfb.org

Emphasis: Offers information on materials, referrals, and job services of interest to the blind.

NAVH Mailing List (National Association for Visually Handicapped)

Computerized administrator: navhmail-request@navh.org

Human administrator: listguide@navh.org

Emphasis: Provides a means for people dealing with vision impairment to share their knowlege and experience on a variety of topics. Open to members of NAVH.

To subscribe: Send e-mail to the computerized administrator. In the body of the message, type: subscribe.

On-Line Connection!'s Disability, Medical, and Health Resources

Web site: www.kansas.net/~cbaslock

Emphasis: Provides information on medical and health-related resources for the disabled.

Prevent Blindness America

Web site: www.prevent-blindness.org

Emphasis: Provides information on vision, eye health, and safety and provides links to other related sites.

Rand Eye Institute

Web site: www.randeye.com

Emphasis: Provides information on the Rand Eye Foundation, which provides eyecare education for the community and continuing education for optometrists and ophthalmologists.

RPLIST List (Retinal degeneration and low-vision discussion list)
Computerized administrator: listserv@maelstrom.stjohns.edu
Human administrator: rplist-request@maelstrom.stjohns.edu
Emphasis: Provides discussion forum.
To subscribe: Send e-mail to computerized administrator. In the body of the message, type: subscribe rplist [your name or the name you want to be known by on the list].

Schepens Eye Research Institute
Harvard Medical School
Web site: www.eri.harvard.edu
Emphasis: Provides information on current research and links to vision-related sites.

SeniorCom
Web site: www.senior.com
Emphasis: Provides age-related resources, with a special focus on health and wellness.

SeniorLink
Web site: www.seniorlink.com
Emphasis: Serves as a national eldercare resource, referral, and consultation Web site for seniors, their families, and providers.

SeniorNet
Web site: www.seniornet.org
Emphasis: Provides seniors with information and instruction about computer technologies; sponsors SeniorNet Learning Centers; publishes computer-related materials; holds national conferences and conducts research on the uses of technology by older adults.

Seniors-site
Web site: www.seniors-site.com/
Emphasis: Provides information and links to other Web sites of interest to senior citizens.

Sight and Hearing Association

Web site: www.sightandhearing.org

Emphasis: Provides information on the prevention of loss of vision and hearing.

Telesensory

Web site: www.telesensory.com

Emphasis: Sells high-tech vision-related equipment and products, including internet browsers.

Third Age

Web site: www.thirdage.com

Emphasis: Provides information and links to resources of interest to adults.

Vision Enhancement

Vision Worldwide

Web site: www.netdirect.net/vision-enhancement

Emphasis: Provides information and referrals in a variety of media for individuals and professionals concerned with vision loss (speech-friendly site).

Vision Rehab Centers

Web site: www.visionrehab.com

Emphasis: Provides information on low-vision care and devices, as well as links to related sites.

Visual Health and Surgical Center

Columbia Healthcare Corporation

Web site: www.web-xpress.com/vhsc

Emphasis: Provides information on visual health and treatment for eye conditions and diseases.

Washington Assistive Technology Alliance

Web site: www.wata.org

Emphasis: Provides referrals for funding and sources for assistive technology.

Notes

Chapter 2

"Age-Related Macular Degeneration." Prevent Blindness America, 1995.

"Macular Degeneration: What It Is, What Causes It, What Can Be Done." The Lighthouse, May 1996.

Chapter 3

AARP Bulletin. American Association of Retired Persons, Vol. 39, No. 1, January 1998.

The McIntyre Report. McIntyre Eye Clinic and Surgical Center, Vol. XIV, Winter 1998.

"Tips for Talking with Your Doctor." National Eye Institute, National Institutes of Health, NIH Publication No. 96-4032, July 3, 1997.

Chapter 4

"A Cautious Comeback for Thalidomide." *Harvard Health Letter,* February 1998, p. 5.

Adler, Tina. "Researchers Spot Another Blinding Gene." *Science News,* December 3, 1994, p. 374.

Cooke, Robert. "Testing Finds Gene Causing Blindness." *Seattle Times,* September 19, 1997, p. 11.

"Dog Blindness Has Genetic Link to Human Form." Cornell University and the Fred Hutchison Cancer Research Center, Top Stories Headlines, March 17, 1998.

Feldman, Miriam K. "ARMD Radiation Study Raises Hope—Unreasonably?" *Argus News Magazine,* March 1997.

Grady, Denise. "Gene Discovery May Lead to Test for Devastating Eye Disorder." *New York Times,* March 4, 1997.

"How Is Macular Degeneration Diagnosed?" *The Magnifier,* Macular Degeneration Foundation, Volume 1, Spring 1994.

Kahn, Carol. "How to Improve Your Eyesight." *Parade* magazine, September 13, 1998, p. 20.

Lubell, Deann. "Age-related Macular Degeneration: When Things Don't Look Sharp, It's Time to Have Your Eyes Checked." *Desert Sun,* December 21, 1997.

"Macular Degeneration: What It Is, What Causes It, What Can Be Done." The Lighthouse, May 1996.

"Miravant Announces 1997 Results." Miravant press release, March 12, 1998.

"More Research Focusing on AMD: Cause, Treatment, and Prevention Getting Attention." *Prism.* Community Services for the Blind and Partially Sighted, Spring 1998, p. 1.

" 'Pain-free' Macular Degeneration Drug in Final Trials Before Seeking Approval." *97 Aging News Alert,* CD publications staff, no date.

"Prescription for Independence." American Foundation for the Blind, no date.

"Research to Detect and Correct AMD." *The Magnifier,* Macular Degeneration Foundation, Vol. 2, Fall 1994.

Stone, Edwin. "What We Need to Find Is a $1 Solution. . . ." University of Iowa Hospitals and Clinics, no date.

"Valuable Vices: Researcher Uncovers the Healthful Side of Hedonism." *Science News,* Vol. 153, February 28, 1998, p. 142.

Chapter 5

Loveren, Nancy. Center for Continuing Education and Rehabilitation. Interview by author, Seattle, April 1998.

"Low Vision Questions and Answers: Definitions, Devices, Services." American Foundation for the Blind, no date.

Rubin, Stanford, and Richard Roessler. *Foundations of the Vocational Rehabilitation Process.* Baltimore: University Park Press, 1978, pp. 19–45.

Seattle Lighthouse Project. Tour by the author, Fall 1997.

"That All May Read." Library Service for Blind and Physically Handicapped People, Library of Congress, 1983.

Washington Talking Books and Braille Library. Tour by the author with Phyllis Cairns, March 12, 1998.

Chapter 6

"Aging and Vision: Making the Most of Impaired Vision." American Association of Retired Persons and American Foundation for the Blind, 1987.

Dayhoff, Tina. "Ask Enough Questions, and Someone's Bound to Answer." *Fighting Blindness News,* Foundation Fighting Blindness, September 1996.

Levner, Henrietta. "I Keep Five Pair of Glasses in a Flower Pot." National Association for the Visually Handicapped, 1985.

The Lighthouse 1997 catalog.

LS&S Group 1998 catalog.

"Macular Degeneration: What It Is, What Causes It, What Can Be Done." The Lighthouse, May 1996.

"Making the World More Accessible." Community Services for the Blind and Partially Sighted, Adaptive Aids and Technology Store, 1997 catalog.

Maxi-Aids and Appliances 1997–98 catalog.

"Questions and Answers About Optical Devices." Lighthouse National Center for Vision and Aging, no date.

"Tips for Home and Travel." American Foundation for the Blind, no date.

"Tips for Living with AMD." Prevent Blindness America, 1995.

"Visual Impairment and Blindness: A Resource Guide." Community Services for the Blind and Partially Sighted, 6th ed., no date.

Chapter 7

Applegate, Martha. Community Services for the Blind and Partially Sighted. Interview by author, April 1998.

Arlene R. Gordon Research Institute. "The Role of Personality Traits and Coping Strategies in Late-Life Adaptation to Vision Loss." The Lighthouse, no date.

Bartlett, John. *Bartlett's Familiar Quotations.* Boston: Little, Brown and Company, 1980.

"Emotional Aspects of Vision Loss." *Prism.* Community Services for the Blind and Partially Sighted, Winter 1996.

Gallup, M.A., Carol. "Better Vision, Healthier Eyes." *New Times,* January 1998.

Hinton, Dr. Ladson. Interview by author, Seattle, February 1998.

"Macular Degeneration: What It Is, What Causes It, What Can Be Done." The Lighthouse, May 1996.

"Sharing Solutions." New York: Lighthouse National Center for Vision and Aging, Spring 1997.

Chapter 8

American Academy of Ophthalmology, San Francisco.

Baker, Beth. "Anti-Aging Humbug: There's No Magic Bullet." *AARP Bulletin,* Vol. 38, No. 4, April 1997.

Balch, Phyllis A., and James F. Balch. *Prescription for Nutritional Healing.* Garden City Park, NY: Avery Publishing Group, 1996.

"Experts Caution to Be Aware of Risk in Some Dietary Supplements." *Methow Valley News,* April 9, 1998.

Gallup, M.A., Carol. "Better Vision, Healthier Eyes." *New Times,* January 1998.

Giller, Robert, MD. *Natural Prescriptions.* New York: Carol Southern Books, 1994.

Golan, Ralph. *Optimal Wellness.* New York: Ballantine Books, 1995.

"Macular Degeneration: What It Is, What Causes It, What Can Be Done." The Lighthouse, May 1996.

Mitchell, Bill. Interview with the author, Seattle, April 1998.

Ody, Penelope. *The Complete Medicinal Herbal: A Practical Guide to the Healing Properties of Herbs.* London: Dorling Kindersley, 1993.

Ronzio, Robert. *Encyclopedia of Nutrition and Good Health,* New York: Facts on File, 1997.

Science News, Vol. 153, February 28, 1998, p. 142.

Somer, Elizabeth. *Essential Guide to Vitamins and Minerals: Everything You Need to Know to Improve Your Diet, Nutrition, and Health.* New York: Harper Collins, 1992.

"Supplements Are Not Regulated by the Government." *Eyes Only.* Association for Macular Diseases, Winter 1998.

"Voice of the British Macular Society." British Macular Society, July 1996.

Weil, Andrew, MD. *Eight Weeks to Optimum Health: A Proven Program for Taking Full Advantage of Your Body's Natural Healing Power*. New York: Alfred A. Knopf, 1997.

Chapter 9

"The Lighthouse National Survey on Vision Loss: The Experience, Attitudes, and Knowledge of Middle-Aged and Older Americans." The Lighthouse, 1996.

Chapter 10

Alliance for Technology Access. *Computer Resources for People with Disabilities: A Guide to Exploring Today's Assistive Technology*. Alameda, CA: Hunter House, 1996.

The Lighthouse 1997 catalog.

LS&S Group 1998 catalog.

Maxi-Aids and Appliances 1997–98 catalog.

National Institutes of Health, University of Utah, Johns Hopkins Medical School, University of Bonn in Germany, January 2, 1998.

Prism, Vol. 5, No. 4. Community Services for the Blind and Partially Sighted, Winter 1997.

Wu, Corinna. "Supernatural Vision: A Focus on Adaptive Optics Improves Images of the Eye and Boosts Vision." *Science News,* Vol. 152, November 15, 1997, p. 312.

Chapter 11

"Audio-described Movies, Theater, and Disabled Sports USA." *Prism,* Community Services for the Blind and Partially Sighted, Spring 1998.

Washington Talking Books and Braille Library. Author tour, March 1998.

Chapter 12

All personal stories in this chapter and throughout the book have been culled from author correspondence and conversations with people during 1997 and 1998.

Glossary

Age-related Macular Degeneration (AMD) — A form of macular degeneration that occurs generally among those 45 and older.

Amsler Grid — A network or pattern of lines used in eye testing to detect distortions or defects in vision.

Antioxidants — Naturally occurring chemicals that assist the body in preventing and arresting some ailments known to affect the aging population.

Astigmatism — Refractive distortion usually due to a change in the curvature of the eyes: the cornea and lens.

Atrophic Macular Degeneration — A dry form of macular degeneration in which cells waste away or die in one area of the macula.

Blood Spots — Spots of blood on the eye's retina that are visible only through an ophthalmoscope and can be a symptom of eye disease.

Books on Tape — *See* Talking Books.

Cameo — As used by the author, a brief profile of those interviewed for this book, signified in the text by a cameo symbol.

Cataract — An eye disease occurring as cells collect inside the interior lens of the eye, causing it to cloud up.

CCTV — *See* Closed-Circuit Television.

Central (Direct) Vision — The area of vision directly in front of the eyes—what a person is looking right at.

Closed-Circuit Television (CCTV) — A desktop magnifier capable of enlarging text up to 60 times normal size.

Cones — Light-sensitive retinal cells that facilitate sharp vision in bright light and color discrimination.

Cornea — The transparent skin and the eye's outermost lens that collects and directs light into the eye.

Descriptive Video Services (DVS) — Audio service of narration of key visual elements and action available with many television programs and videos.

Dry Macular Degeneration — Any of the forms of central retina damage that do not feature leakage of blood or liquid into or under the retina. *See also* Atrophic Macular Degeneration.

Far-Sightedness (Hyperopia) — A diminished ability to see (unless corrected by lenses) objects that are near, a form of refractive error.

Fluorescein Angiogram — A procedure in which a dye is injected into a patient's bloodstream, allowing any abnormal blood vessel hemorrhages in the eye to be seen with a special camera.

Fovea Centralis — Central pit in the macula that contains a high concentration of cones, producing the sharpest vision.

Free Radicals — Destructive molecules in the tissues of the body, usually the result of oxidation.

Glaucoma — An eye condition that can cause blindness due to excessive fluid pressure within the eye.

Hallucination — Condition where shapes seem to appear in the visual field but do not actually exist even though they seem real to the affected person.

Halogen lamps — Lamps that use halogen bulbs, which produce bright light without glare.

Iris — The colored membrane surrounding the pupil suspended between the eye's lens and the cornea.

Juvenile Macular Degeneration — A variation of macular degeneration with a strong hereditary component (sometimes called Stargardt disease) that occurs in young people.

Laser Therapy — A treatment in which a beam of light is used to sear tissues of the eye.

Legal Blindness — Condition of sight when a person's best corrected central visual acuity is 20/200 or worse in the better eye, or periphery (side vision) is narrowed to 20 degrees or less.

Low Vision (LV) — Usable vision that is imperfect and cannot be fully corrected by ordinary glasses, medical treatment, or surgery. Examples of low vision include overall blurred vision, loss of central vision, and loss of peripheral vision.

Low-Vision Clinic — A medical clinic specializing in treating clients with low vision. Most also carry products designed for the visually impaired.

Macula — The small area at the very back of the retina, in the center of the eye, that clarifies small details in direct vision.

Macular Degeneration — An incurable (at least at this writing) eye disease caused by a breakdown of cells and tissues in the macula and in some cases abnormal blood vessel growth or leakage around the retina.

Naturopathic Doctor (ND) — A general practitioner, not necessarily a medical doctor, whose training encompasses a broad spectrum of natural therapies, as well as the standard health sciences.

Near-Sightedness (Myopia) — The diminished ability to see objects far away, a form of refractive error.

Ophthalmologist — A medical doctor (MD) who specializes in the treatment of eye disorders.

Ophthalmoscope — An instrument for examining the interior of the eye.

Optician — Someone who crafts and fits corrective lenses from prescriptions written by optometrists.

Optometrist — A doctor of optometry (not an MD) who examines the eyes to prescribe lenses that correct the symptoms of refractive disorders such as near- and far-sightedness, and astigmatism.

Oxidation — A chemical reaction that occurs in the body, sometimes destructive. It may be facilitated by light energy.

Partially sighted — One of the various terms given to those who have visual impairment.

Peripheral (Side) Vision — Sight associated with the outer area of the field of vision, away from the center.

Photoreceptors — The rod and cone cells of the retina that are capable of being stimulated by light.

Pupil — The black opening at the center of the iris. The iris muscles control the size of the opening.

Radiation Treatment — A form of treatment used to halt the buildup of abnormal blood vessels or other tissues such as tumors.

Retina — The layer of tissue that lines the inside of the eye and receives the image formed by the lens.

Retinist — A medical doctor (MD) who specializes in the diagnosis and treatment of retinal disorders, which are a subspecialty of ophthalmology, requiring additional "fellowship" training.

Retinitis Pigmentosa (RP) — A group of eye diseases that first affect peripheral vision and can result in blindness depending on the form of the disease.

Risk Factors — Behaviors or traits (such as smoking or heredity) that can increase the probability of developing a health disorder.

Rods — Light-sensitive retinal cells that facilitate vision in dim light and in the periphery.

RP — *See* Retinitis Pigmentosa.

Sclera — The outer skin of the eye, known as the "white of the eye," part of which is visible in the front of the eye.

Services for the Blind — All organizations that assist people with visual impairments.

SHIBA (Senior Health Insurance Benefits Advisors) — Washington state program to train senior volunteers who provide free, impartial, and confidential counsel to their peers on health insurance issues. *See also* Resources.

Sight-disabled — One of the various terms given to those who have visual impairment.

Stargardt Disease — A hereditary eye disease, sometimes called *juvenile macular degeneration,* which is similar to macular degeneration and found in young people.

Subretinal Neovascularization — Occurs in "wet" macular degeneration when blood vessels grow abnormally, causing blood, water, or protein leakage in the retina.

Supplements — Vitamin and mineral products intended to add beneficial nutrients that may be missing or unavailable in one's diet.

Talking Books —Audiotaped books available for rent through the Library of Congress that require the use of special cassette players (provided). Other audiobooks, known as books on tape, are playable on standard cassette decks, and are available commercially and free through public libraries.

Uveitis — A general term for inflammatory diseases inside the eye.

Visual Disability — The attempt to quantify the condition of sight, measured in percentages, wherein a person's level of vision prevents them from performing certain tasks.

Vitreous (vitreous humor, vitreous gel) — The clear gelatinous mass that fills the rear two thirds of the eyeball, between the lens and the retina.

Wet Macular Degeneration — *See* Subretinal Neovascularization.

Index

A

acupressure, 127–129
acupuncture, 108, 127–129
Adair, Virginia, 176–177
adaptive optics, 156
Administration on Aging, 188
AFB Press, 188
Against All Odds, 189
age-related macular degeneration (definition), 232
alcohol and macular degeneration, 48
alternative health care, 36
American Academy of Ophthalmology, 189
American Association of Retired Persons, 36, 189
American Association of the Deaf-Blind, 189
American Bible Society, 190
American Council of the Blind, 190
American Foundation for the Blind, 190
American Macular Degeneration Foundation, 190
American Medical Association, 34
American Printing House for the Blind, 191
Amsler grid, 42, 232
animals, 106
anthocyanoside, 112, 123
antibody drug, 55
antioxidants, 48, 49, 119–121, 232
Arkenstone, 191
art, 105
assistance, finding, 134–145
Associated Services for the Blind, 191
Association for Macular Diseases, 192
Association for Radio Reading Services, 192
Association for the Rehabilitation of the Blind and Visually Impaired, 192

astigmatism, 232
atrophic macular degeneration, see dry macular degeneration
attitude, positive, 175–176, 177–187
Audio Description, 192
Audio Editions, 193
Audio Renaissance, 193

B

B vitamins, 48, 121
banking, 136–137
Bates method, 130–132
Bates, William, 96
bathroom safety, 81–82
berries, 112
Bible Alliance, 193
bilberries, 112, 132
bioflavonoids, 124
Blackstone Audio Books, 193
blind spots, 44
blindness, see macular degeneration
blindness, causes of, 21
blindness, legal, 234
Blindskills, 193
blood spots, 9, 10, 12, 23, 232
blood vessels, 17
blueberries, 112
blurring, 42
books on tape, 162–164, 194
Books on Tape, 194
BPD (benzoporphyrene) drug treatment, 55
Braille Circulating Library, 194
braille libraries, 69–70
brain, 20

C

caffeine and macular degeneration, 48
calculators, talking, 88, 149
Careers and Technology Information Bank, 194

Carolyn's, 194
carotein, 112
carrots, 112, 113, 114
cataracts, 18, 21, 29, 42, 43, 45, 49,
    232; surgery and macular degener-
    ation, 7, 50
Center for Self-Healing, 195
Center for the Partially Sighted, 195
central direct vision, 232
chard, 115
Charles Bonet syndrome, 24
Chivers Audio Books, 195
Choice Magazine Listening, 195
cholesterol, 48, 115
choroid, 19, 23
clocks, talking, 89, 148
closed-circuit televisions, 63–64, 87,
    147–149, 232
colors, faded, 43
Committee for the Medically
    Underserved, 196
Community Services for the Blind and
    Partially Sighted, 60, 196
computer hardware, 38, 50, 152–154
computer monitors, 50
computer screen readers, 38
computer software, 149–152
computers, purchasing, 154
concerts, 161
cone cells, 19, 232
cornea, 17, 18, 233
Council of Citizens with Low Vision
    International, 196
Creative Adaptations for Learning, 196
cruises, 168
cultural festivals, 169

D

dance, 161
DECtalk, 153
Delta Gamma Foundation, 197
depression, 4, 9, 95
Descriptive Video Services, 166–167,
    197, 232

diabetes and macular degeneration,
    47–48, 49
diabetic retinopathy, 2, 30, 42, 43,
    47–48; and laser treatments, 52
diet and macular degeneration, 48
Disabled Sports USA, 171–172
double vision, 43
Doubleday Large Print Home Library,
    197
dreams, 98–100
dry macular degeneration, 51, 232, 233
dry eyes, 42
dyes, 46; see also fluorescein
    angiograms

E

Easier Ways, 197
Educational Tape Recording for the
    Blind, 198
Eldercare Locator, 198
Elderhostel, 168, 198
electronic retinal implants, 56
empathy, medical, 30–33
epiretinal membrane, 43
equipment, 62, 63
exercise, 97, 125–127
Eye Bank Association of America, 198
eye doctors, 28–39; choosing, 33–35
eye examination, self, 44–46
eye exercises, 130–132
eye structure, 17–21
eye, inner, 29; diagram, 17
eyebright (herb), 124
eyeglasses, 41, 59

F

familial exultative maculopathy, 48
far-sightedness, 233
fats, dietary, 48, 115–117
fear, 100–101
fetal cell transplants, 54, 56
fiber, dietary, 49, 117
fire, 79
fish oils, 123–124

floaters, 44
floor safety, 76–77
fluorescein angiogram, 10, 12, 233
Foundation Fighting Blindness, 198
Foundation for Glaucoma Research, 199
Foundation of the American Academy of
    Ophthalmology, 199
fovea centralis, 17, 20, 233
free radicals, 56, 120, 233
friends, 142–143

G

genetic risks, 47–48
genetic treatment and Stargardt dis-
    ease, 54
ginkgo, 122–123
Glaucoma Research Foundation, 199
Glaucoma Support Network, 199
glaucoma, 18, 21, 29, 43, 45, 233
golf, 171
greens, 112
grocery shopping, 135–136

H

hallucinations, 24, 233
halogen lamps, 78, 233
hardware, computer, 38, 50, 152–154
heart disease and macular degenera-
    tion, 49
Helen Keller International, 200
herbs, 108, 122–125
hiking, 171
home safety, 75–91
humor, 32–33
hydrogenated fats, 115
hypertension and macular degenera-
    tion, 49
hysterical blindness, 96

I

ICAPS, 58
In Touch Networks, 200
Independent Living Aids, 200

Institute for Families of Blind Children,
    200
insurance coverage, choosing, 35–37
International Lions Club, 64, 66, 71, 201
Internet, 152; resources, 218–227
iris, 17, 18, 233
iritis, 42, 108
itching, 44

J

Jewish Heritage for the Blind, 201
John Milton Society for the Blind, 201
juvenile macular degeneration, see
    Stargardt disease

K

Keller, Helen, 70–72, 176
keyboard enhancing software, 150
keyboards, computer, 153
King, Stephen, 22
kitchen safety, 79–81
Kiwanis, 139
Kurzweil, 201

L

lamps, 77
large-print books, 213
laser treatments, 32, 51–52, 234
lens, 17, 18
Library of Congress, 69, 169, 201
library resources, 167
light flashes, 43
light sensitivity, 42, 50
Lighthouse Inc., The, 65, 89, 202
lighting, 76–77, 78, 80
Lions Sight Conservation Foundation,
    202
Listening Library, 203
Love Bike, 203
low vision, definition, 234
low-vision clinics, 2, 38, 60–66
low-vision support groups, 2, 203
LS&S Group, 89, 203
lutein, 112, 124

M

macula, 1, 11, 17, 234; function of, 19

macular degeneration, 1, 30, 45; and age, 1, 21–23; and gender, 48; causes of, 22; definition, 11, 234; dry, 22–23, 51, 232, 233; and race, 49; risk factors, 47–51; symptoms, 4–11, 40–46; treatments, 51–58; wet, 12, 22–23, 236

Macular Degeneration Awareness, 204

Macular Degeneration Foundation, 22, 37, 204

Macular Degeneration International, 204

macular dystrophy, 2

magnifiers, 38, 63, 64, 85–87; systems, 147, 148

Massachusetts Association for the Blind, 205

massage, 129

Maxi-Aids, 89, 205

McIntyre Eye Clinic, 11

Medicare, 35, 64

Medigap insurance, 36

meditation, 101–102

Microsoft Guide to Windows 95 Keyboard Commands, 205

milk thistle, 124

Miravent, 55

movie videos, 166–167

multivitamins, 125

music, 103–105, 161–162

N

National Association for Parents of the Visually Impaired, 206

National Association for Visually Handicapped, 206

National Association of Area Agencies on Aging, 206

National Coalition for Deaf-Blindness, 206

National Eye Care Project, 207

National Eye Institute, 207

National Federation of the Blind, 207

National Library Service for the Blind and Physically Handicapped, 69, 162, 163, 208

National Resource Guide, 208

National Retinitis Pigmentosa Foundation, 208

naturopathy, 11, 234

near-sightedness, 234

neurons, 19

New Visions Store, 208

New York Free Circulating Library for the Blind, 72

Newsline for the Blind, 165

Newspapers for the Blind, 208

newspapers, 165

night vision, 44

Nostalgia Television, 209

nutrition, 110–125

O

omega-3 fatty acids, 123–124

OpenBook, 147

ophthalmologists, 29–30, 234

ophthalmoscopes, 46

optic nerve, 17, 18

optical character recognition software, 146, 147, 151–152

opticians, 29, 234

optometrists, 29, 234

oranges, 115

oxidation, 235

P

pain, 43

patient responsibility, 33

performing arts, 167–168

peripheral vision, 43–44, 235

pets, 106

PhotoPoint treatment, 55

photoreceptors, 19, 235

pigment epithelium detachment, 37

plasmapheresis, 53

pot marigold (herb), 124
prayer, 102–103
Prevent Blindness America, 209
pupil, 17, 18, 235

R

race and macular degeneration, 49
radiation treatment, 13–17, 23–24, 53, 235
radio, 164–166
Randolph-Shepard Act, 72
RDAs, 119
recipes, tofu, 116–117; vitamin A, 113–114
Recorded Books, 210
Recording for the Blind, 210
recreation, 160–174
reflexology, 129–130
rehabilitation training, 63, 66, 68–69
relaxation, 103, 105–106
Resources for Rehabilitation, 210
resources, 59–74
Retina Research Fund, 210
retina, 1, 11, 17, 18, 235
retinal cell transplant, 54
retinal detachment, 42, 44
retinal implant system, 155
retinal pigment epithelium cells, 19, 23, 54
retinal repositioning, 54
retinists, 29, 30
retinitis pigmentosa, 2, 24–25, 30, 44, 47, 235; and genetic links, 54
RheoTherapy, 53
rod cells, 19, 235
Rotary Club, 139
RP Foundation Fighting Blindness, 211

S

safety, home, 75–91
SAP radio programming, 164–165
saturated fats, 115
scanner, 147
scanning laser opthalmoscope, 46

Schepens Eye Research Institute, 211
sclera, 17, 18, 19, 235
screen enlarging software, 150–151
screen translating software, 151
seating, 78–79
Seattle Lighthouse Project, 66–67
seaweed, 122
seitan, 116
selenium, 120, 124
Senior Health Insurance Benefits Advisors, 236
Seniors Helping Seniors, 34, 36
Sight First, 71
singing, 161
skiing, 171
Social Security Administration, 211
software, 149–152
software, reading, 146–147
software, voice synthesizer, 146–147
Spectrum, 211
spinach, 114
sports, 170–172
stairs, 77
Stargardt disease, 1, 26–27, 37, 38, 233, 236; genetic links, 47; genetic treatment for, 54
State Department of Services for the Blind, 212
State Rehabilitation Agency, 212
State School for the Blind, 212
state services for the blind, 65, 67–69
stationary night blindness, 48
Sticker's syndrome, 48
stress, 9, 11, 43; physical effects of, 92–97; prevention, 97–98; relieving, 97–109
stroke and macular degeneration, 15, 44, 49
Strontium-90 treatment, 55
subretinal neovascularization, see wet macular degeneration
sugar, 48
Sullivan, Annie, 71
sunlight, 49

support groups, 140–142
suspensory ligament, 17

T

tai chi, 126–127
Talking Books Library, 162, 163
talking books, 4, 69–70, 162–164
Taping for the Blind, 213
taste, sense of, 170
taxes, 137
telephone service, 137
telephone tips, 84–85
Telesensory, 213
text translation software, 153
thalidomide, 56
Thorndike Press, 213
tobacco and macular degeneration, 48
tofu, 116
touch, sense of, 169–170
transportation, 34, 137–138
travel, 168–169
turmeric, 124

U

U.S. Blind Golfers Association, 171
ultrasound, 46
ultraviolet rays, exposure to, 49
uveitis, 73, 108, 236

V

vascular endothelial growth factor, 55
vegetables, 112
virtual retinal display, 56, 154–155
VISION Foundation, 213
Vision Rehab Centers, 214
vision problems, symptoms of macular
    degeneration, 41–44
vision, night, 44
VISIONS/Services for the Blind and
    Visually Impaired, 214
vitamin A, 48, 112, 120; recipes rich
    in, 113–114
vitamin B, 48, 112

vitamin C, 119, 120, 121
vitamin E, 120, 121
vitamin supplements, 48, 118–122
vitreous humor, 17, 18, 236
V-max, 148
voice recognition software, 151
voice synthesizers, 146–148
Voices of Vision, 163
volunteers, 138–140

W

walking stick, 87–88
walking, 125–126
Washington Assistive Technology
    Alliance, 214
Washington Talking Books and Braille
    Library, 69–70
watches, talking, 148
water, 112, 13
wavy lines, 42
wet macular degeneration, 12, 13, 22–
    23, 236; laser treatments, 52; radi-
    ation treatments, 53; treatment
    of, 55
wine, red, 48
women and macular degeneration, 48
World at Large, 215
wristwatches, 89

X

xanthophyll, 112
Xavier Society for the Blind, 215
Xerox Imaging Systems, 215

Y

yams, 114
yoga, 126–127
yogurt, 112

Z

zeaxanthin, 123
zinc, 48, 122

CANCER

CANCER—INCREASING YOUR ODDS FOR SURVIVAL: A Resource Guide for Integrating Mainstream, Alternative and Complementary Therapies
by David Bognar

Based on the four-part public television series hosted by Walter Cronkite.

This book provides cancer patients and their families a comprehensive look at traditional medical treatments and how these can be supplemented with healing techniques and support methods that have been shown to work. The book explains the basics of cancer and the best actions to take immediately after a diagnosis of cancer. It outlines the various treatments — conventional, alternative, and complementary; describes the powerful effect the mind can have on the body and the therapies that strengthen this connection; and explores spiritual healing and issues surrounding death and dying. Includes full-length interviews with leaders in the field of healing, including Joan Borysenko, Lawrence LeShan, Stephen Levine, and Bernie Siegel.

320 pages ... Paperback $15.95 ... Hard cover $25.95

CANCER DOESN'T HAVE TO HURT: How to Conquer the Pain Caused by Cancer and Cancer Treatment
by Pamela J. Haylock, R.N., and Carol P. Curtiss, R.N.

People with cancer often suffer needlessly because of the belief that cancer and pain go hand in hand. Two respected cancer nurses show that not only can cancer's pain be relieved, but patients whose pain is eased live longer, healthier cancer patients and their families find and pay for effective pain control. Haylock and Curtiss each have more than 20 years of experience and use careful, direct language to detail pain management options including opiates, non-opiates, and the controversial use of marijuana. Readers learn how to describe their pain in specific terms that doctors understand, as well as how to read prescriptions, administer medications, and adjust dosages, if necessary. The book offers non-drug methods of pain relief that patients and caregivers can implement on their own, including massage, exercise, visual imagery, and music therapy.

192 pages ... 12 illus. ... Paperback $14.95 ... Hard cover $24.95

RECOVERING FROM BREAST SURGERY: Exercises to Strengthen Your Body and Relieve Pain *by* Diana Stumm, P.T.

Many women find that breast surgery leaves them with crippling pain. Until now, no book has specifically addressed how to eliminate the pain that follows a mastectomy or breast surgery. Physical therapist Diana Stumm has worked with women recovering from breast surgery for many years and in this book explains how to recuperate and recover mobility. With warmth and understanding, she discusses the best exercises for mastectomy, lumpectomy, radiation, reconstruction, and lymphedema. Using clear drawings, she describes a program of specific stretches, massage techniques, and general exercises that form the crucial steps to a full and pain-free recovery.

128 pages ... 25 illus. ... Paperback ... $11.95

To order books or a FREE catalog see last page or call (800) 266-5592

WOMEN'S HEALTH

MENOPAUSE WITHOUT MEDICINE *by* Linda Ojeda, Ph.D.

Amidst all the hype about menopause, there is a greater need than ever for accurate information and guidelines for effective self-care. This book, by a renowned author and health educator, gives women the well-researched advice they need to approach menopause naturally and positively. Linda Ojeda broke new ground when she began her study of nonmedical approaches to menopause more than ten years ago. Now she has fully updated her classic book. She discusses natural sources of estrogen, including phytoestrogens; how mood swings are affected by diet and personality; and the newest research on osteoporosis, breast cancer, and heart disease. She thoroughly examines the hormone therapy debate; suggests natural remedies for depression, hot flashes, sexual changes, and skin and hair problems; and presents an illustrated basic exercise program. Ojeda shows how women can enjoy optimal health at any age with a good diet and nurturing lifestyle. As seen in *Time* magazine.

352 pages ... 40 illus. ... Paperback $14.95 ... Hard cover $23.95 ... 3rd edition

HER HEALTHY HEART: A Woman's Guide to Preventing and Reversing Heart Disease Naturally *by* Linda Ojeda, Ph.D.

Heart disease is the #1 killer of women ages 44 to 65, yet up until now most of the research and attention has been given to men. This book fills this gap by addressing the unique aspects of heart disease in women and the natural ways to combat it. Dr. Linda Ojeda explains how women can prevent heart disease whether they take hormone replacement therapy (HRT) or not. She also provides detailed information on how women can reduce their risk of heart disease by making changes in diet, increasing physical activity, and managing stress. A 50-item lifestyle questionnaire is included to help women evaluate their current physical and emotional health and pinpoint areas to work on.

352 pages ... 12 illus. ... Paperback $14.95

THE NATURAL ESTROGEN DIET: Healthy Recipes for Perimenopause and Menopause *by* Dr. Lana Liew with Linda Ojeda, Ph.D.

To manage the symptoms of menopause, doctors are prescribing hormone replacement therapy (HRT) at record levels. Recent studies, however, show that increasing the natural estrogen in the diet can successfully manage menopause.

Here, two women's health and nutrition experts offer women more than 100 easy and delicious recipes to naturally increase their level of estrogen. Each recipe includes nutritional information such as the calories, cholesterol, and calcium content. The authors also provide an overview of how phytoestrogens (plant estrogen) work, which foods contain the highest levels of natural estrogen, and how to approach a natural estrogen diet successfully. A general health plan for women forms an important part of the book emphasizing preventative measures and encouraging good health practices.

192 pages ... 25 illus. ... Paperback $13.95

To order books or a FREE catalog see last page or call (800) 266-5592

GENERAL HEALTH

FAD-FREE NUTRITION *by* Fredrick J. Stare, M.D., Ph.D., and Elizabeth M. Whelan, Sc.D., M.P.H.

The media is flooded with claims of quick-fix nutritional nirvanas. Using up-to-date nutrition information and basing their approach on sound scientific principles and legitimate studies, the authors help the reader sort fact from fiction. They debunk claims that the food supply is irreversibly tainted, that disease is an inevitable result of eating, that nutritional supplements are a necessity, and that food technology is employed against the public interest.

Fredrick J. Stare, M.D., Ph.D., founded the Department of Nutrition at Harvard University's School of Public Health in 1942. **Elizabeth M. Whelan, Sc.D., M.P.H.,** is president and a founder of the American Council on Science and Health.

256 pages ... Paperback ... $14.95

TREAT YOUR BACK WITHOUT SURGERY: The Best Non-Surgical Alternatives for Eliminating Back and Neck Pain *by* Stephen Hochschuler, M.D., and Bob Reznik

Eighty percent of back pain sufferers can get well without surgery. Be one of them! From the authors of *Back in Shape,* this new guide discusses a range of non-surgical techniques — from Tai Chi and massage therapy to chiropractic treatment and acupuncture — as well as exercise plans, diet and stress management techniques, and tips to ease everyday pain. Because surgery is sometimes necessary, you'll also get advice on how to find the best surgeon and what questions to ask.

224 pages ... 52 illus. ... Paperback $14.95

THE PLEASURE PRESCRIPTION: To Love, to Work, to Play — Life in the Balance *by* Paul Pearsall, Ph.D.   New York Times Bestseller!

This bestselling book is a prescription for stressed-out lives. Dr. Pearsall maintains that contentment, wellness, and long life can be found by devoting time to family, helping others, and slowing down to savor life's pleasures.

Current wisdom suggests that anything that tastes, smells, or feels good can't be good for us. "That's plain wrong," says Dr. Pearsall, a leading proponent of the relationship between pleasure, stress, the immune system, and brain chemistry. "Balanced pleasure is the natural way to physical and mental health."

The Pleasure Prescription makes the connections between physiological research and "Oceanic" wisdom. The Polynesian way is based on enjoying life and connecting with others. Balance, happiness, and health are achieved through the daily practice of the five qualities of "Aloha": patience, connection, pleasantness, modesty, and tenderness. This practice extends to all aspects of life — from loving relationships, parenting, and work, to healing ourselves and caring for our community and planet.

"This book will save your life." — Montel Williams

288 pages ... Paperback $13.95 ... Hard cover $23.95 ... Audio $16.95

Prices subject to change

ORDER FORM

NAME

ADDRESS

CITY/STATE   ZIP/POSTCODE

PHONE   COUNTRY

TITLE	QTY	PRICE	TOTAL
Macular Degeneration		@ $14.95	
Cancer —Increasing Your Odds		@ $15.95	
Cancer Doesn't Have to Hurt		@ $14.95	

Prices subject to change without notice

Please list other titles below:

		@ $	
		@ $	
		@ $	
		@ $	
		@ $	
		@ $	

Shipping costs
First book: $3.00 by book post; $4.50 by UPS or Priority Mail, or to ship outside the U.S.
Each additional book: $1.00
For rush orders and bulk shipments call us at (800) 266-5592

SUBTOTAL	
Less discount @ _____ %	( )
TOTAL COST OF BOOKS	
Calif. residents add sales tax	
Shipping & handling	
TOTAL ENCLOSED	

Please pay in U.S. funds only

❑ Check ❑ Money Order ❑ Visa ❑ M/C ❑ Discover

Card # _____ Exp date _____

Signature _____

Complete and mail to:
Hunter House Inc., Publishers
PO Box 2914, Alameda CA 94501-0914
Orders: 1-800-266-5592 . . . ordering@hunterhouse.com
Phone (510) 865-5282 Fax (510) 865-4295
❑ Check here to receive our FREE book catalog

MAC 9/98